Succeeding in AKT (Applied Knowledge Test) – 500 SBAs, EMQs and Picture MCQs, with a full Mock Test

Chirag Mehta, Mark Williams & Milan Mehta

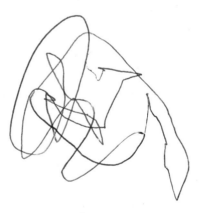

develop
medica

Published by Developmedica
Castle Court
Duke Street
New Basford,
Nottingham, NG7 7JN
0845 838 0571
www.developmedica.com

© 2009 Developmedica

Developmedica recommend that you consult the GP Recruitment website regarding your nMRCGP AKT. The views expressed in this book are those of Developmedica and not those of Royal College of General Practioners and Developmedica are in no way associated with the Royal College of General Practioners or Pearson Vue.

The contents of this book are intended as a guide only and although every effort has been made to ensure that the contents of this book are correct, Developmedica cannot be held responsible for the outcome of any loss or damage that arises through the use of this guide. Readers are advised to seek independent advice regarding their nMRCGP AKT.

Warning: The contents of this revision guide are for the purposes of aiding you to prepare for your nMRCGP AKT only and are not intended to replace the protocols of your current employer.

Every effort has been made to contact the copyright holders of any material reproduced within this publication. If any have been inadvertently overlooked, the publishers will be pleased to make restitution at the earliest opportunity.

A catalogue record for this title is available from the British Library

ISBN: 978-1-906839-10-9

Typeset by Replika Press Pvt. Ltd. (India)

Printed by Bell & Bain, Glasgow

1 2 3 4 5 6 7 8 9 10

Contents

Foreword

Doctors are good at passing exams. That is how we all got to where we are.

But assessment in general practice, as in all the specialties, has moved on. Multiple choice questions have undergone subtle changes and the applied knowledge test (AKT) for Membership of the Royal College of General Practitioners is a different sort of exam. Candidates are not asked to demonstrate knowledge but to apply it.

The computer-based, multi-centre AKT was offered for the sixth time in April 2009. 1102 candidates sat the exam and their mean score was 143 out of 199 questions, with the best candidate scoring 183. 83.8% of candidates passed. Thus bright, well motivated learners are doing well - especially if you sit the exam later on in your training period.

The answers on how to pass the exam will not be found in this book. They will be found during your time in practice seeing lots of patients, focussing on those 'awkward moments' when you realise your training so far has left you completely unprepared for the worries of the patient in front of you. Looking things up in response to patients' unmet needs or doctor's educational needs, talking to your trainer and colleagues, discussing issues that are important to patients and reading widely will get you through the exam. Such is the alignment between this exam and practice that that is also how you will get to be a good GP.

What this book will give you is a way of self-assessing your areas of weakness, showing you where to focus your reading and getting you to think about the breadth and depth of the RCGP curriculum. You won't see everything in practice, rare but important conditions are also part of this exam and you may need reminding of those.

The authors are all trainees who have recently passed the AKT. They have worked hard to develop something that can act as a signpost for you, based on their experience. This book is an excellent jumping off point for your reading.

Good luck!

Kay Mohanna
Chair, RCGP Midland Faculty and Director of Postgraduate Medicine, Keele University.

About the authors

Chirag Mehta is a GP trainee in the West Midland Deanery who qualified from Manchester University in 2006. He has had articles published in the *British Medical Journal*, the GP trainee journal *InnovAit* and also in the journal *Public Health*. He has recently passed his nMRCGP AKT exam in April 2009.

Milan Mehta has come to the end of his GP vocational training within the West Midlands Deanery and has successfully obtained his nMRCGP qualification. He has had articles published in a number of international medical journals and will shortly be taking up a Teaching Fellow post in academic General Practice at Keele University. Together with this he will also continue to work as a part-time salaried GP in Staffordshire.

Mark Williams is a GP trainee who has previously co-authored a book on medical careers, 'The Medical Student Career Handbook' and has had articles published in the *British Medical Journal* and *Emergency Medical Journal*. He has recently passed the nMRCGP AKT.

About the publisher

Developmedica is a specialist provider of books, courses and eLearning solutions tailored to meet your career development needs. Visit our web site at www.developmedica.com and find out more.

Our approach is friendly and personal, and we are only a phone call or an email away.

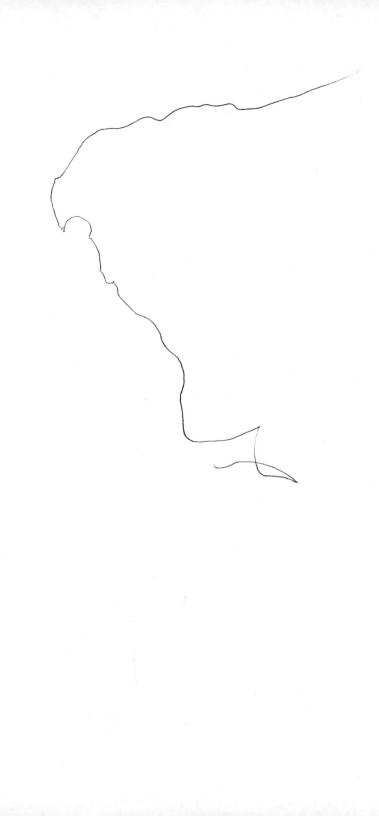

Acknowledgements

We would like to thank Dr Sarah Gear (GP) for her assistance in reviewing the book. We would also like to thank Dr Kay Mohana (Chair of the RCGP Midland Faculty) for writing the foreword for the book. We are also very grateful to Matt Green and his team at Developmedica.

The dermatology pictures Figure 2, Figure 3, Figure 8, Figure 10, Figure 12, Figure 16 and Figure 25 are from © Ashton, Richard and Leppard, Barbara, Differential Diagnosis in Dermatology 3rd edition. Oxford: Radcliffe Publishing; 2005. Reproduced with the permission of the copyright holder.

The ophthalmology pictures Figure 18, Figure 19, Figure 21, Figure 23, Figure 28, Figure 31 are reproduced with permission from James B, Chew C and Bron A (2007) Lecture notes Ophthalmology (10e). Blackwell Publishing.

We would also like to thank the National Institute for Clinical Excellence for allowing us to adapt their tables and algorithms that we have used in Figure 1, Figure 6, Table 4, Figure 24, Figure 45.

National Institute for Clinical Excellence (2003) Adapted from *CG 5 Chronic heart failure: management of chronic heart failure in adults in primary and secondary care*. London: NICE. Available from www.nice.org.uk/CG5 Reproduced with permission.

National Institute for Health and Clinical Excellence (2005) Adapted from *CG 30 Long-acting reversible contraception*. London: NICE. Available from www.nice.org.uk/CG30 Reproduced with permission.

National Institute for Health and Clinical Excellence (2006) Adapted from *CG 34 Hypertension: the management of hypertension in adults in primary care*. London: NICE. Available from www.nice.org.uk/CG34 Reproduced with permission.

National Institute for Health and Clinical Excellence (2007) Adapted from

CG 44 Heavy menstrual bleeding. London: NICE. Available from www. nice.org.uk/CG44 Reproduced with permission.

National Institute for Health and Clinical Excellence (2008) Adapted from *CG 73 Chronic kidney disease: early identification and management of chronic kidney disease in adults in primary and secondary care.* London: NICE. Available from www.nice.org.uk/CG73 Reproduced with permission.

Preface

We are three GP trainees working in Stoke-on-Trent. We have all passed our AKT, and having been through the experience successfully we wanted to write a book to help fellow trainees prepare for it too.

In this book 100 Single Best Answer questions, 100 Extended Match questions and 100 Picture and data interpretation questions allow you to assess yourself and identify areas on which to concentrate your study. When you feel ready, you can go on to take our full 200-question Mock Test under timed conditions; and we believe that this will help prepare you well for the real thing.

We have covered the nMRCGP curriculum throughout and feel that the five hundred questions you will find in this book reflect the challenge you will encounter in the real Test.

A comprehensive Answers section following each set of questions explains the answers clearly. The comprehensive answers to questions plus the helpful references to further reading mean that this book is an effective revision tool.

At the back we have a subject index, so that you can choose to do questions by subject.

We hope that you find this book useful and we wish you all the best for the AKT and the rest of your training.

About the exam and tips on passing it

All trainees now have to sit the nMRCGP examinations in order to qualify as a GP. The Applied Knowledge Test is one of the examinations that GP trainees need to do in order to obtain their nMRCGP. It is a summative assessment of knowledge based upon the RCGP curriculum. Candidates who pass this assessment will have demonstrated their competence in applying knowledge and interpreting information at a level which is sufficiently high for independent practice.

Candidates are able to sit the AKT at any point during their time in GP specialty training.

Format of the test

The test is a 3 hour long paper consisting of 200 questions. It is computer based and is taken at Pearson VUE professional testing centres, of which there are 150 around the UK. It is offered three times a year.

The questions consist of single best answers, extended matching questions and algorithms, data interpretation, diagram, tables and picture questions. Approximately 80% of questions will be on clinical medicine, 10% on critical appraisal and evidence based clinical practice and 10% on health informatics and administrative issues.

The single best answer questions often use a clinical scenario and only one answer is correct. The other options may be plausible and so they ask what is the SINGLE MOST appropriate option.

The extended matching questions have a list of possible options for the theme and there will be several scenarios. The candidate needs to select the most appropriate option that best matches the scenario and each option can be used once, more than once or not at all.

The picture/algorithm/data interpretation questions involve selecting the most appropriate option depending upon the question.

1102 candidates sat the AKT in April 2009. Their mean score was 143 out of 199 scored questions, with the best candidate gaining 183. The pass mark for this exam was set at 126 marks or 63.3%. This resulted in a pass rate of 83.8% for all those candidates taking the test.

The mean scores by subject area were:

- 'Clinical medicine' 74%
- 'Evidence interpretation' 68.2%
- 'Administration questions' 60.1%

There were gaps in knowledge in curriculum statement 8: care of children and young people. The report from the RCGP website on the AKT April 2009 said that items testing the management of childhood asthma were not well answered. Questions from curriculum statement 10: gender specific health issues such as breast disorders were not well answered. Nor were questions around fitness to drive and work (these do fall under curriculum statement 15: clinical management and are important generic issues). Curriculum statement 7: care of acutely ill people had questions on less common potentially life saving procedures which candidates struggled to answer appropriately.

Preparation

Start to prepare early for the exam once you know when you are planning to sit it. We recommend **that you prepare around three months prior to the exam date**. Make sure you have familiarised yourself with the RCGP curriculum and that you read up on any areas you highlight as gaps in your knowledge. There are also many revision sites that are available so you may find these helpful.

We suggest that you look at the following resources:

- Oxford Handbook of General Practice
- Oxford Handbook of Clinical Medicine
- Oxford Handbook of Clinical Surgery
- British National Formulary (BNF)
- Clinical evidence

- Clinical knowledge summaries
- Drug and Therapeutics Bulletin
- British Medical Journal
- Journal of Royal College of General Practitioners
- Innovait
- www.rcgp.org.uk
- www.nice.org.uk
- www.sign.ac.uk
- www.bnf.org.uk
- www.dh.gov.uk
- www.gpnotebook.co.uk
- www.rcog.org.uk
- www.ffprhc.org.uk
- www.bashh.org.uk
- www.dvla.gov.uk
- www.eguidelines.co.uk

Other helpful advice:

- Make a time table of what you need to revise. Your e-portfolio can be used to help you.
- Short periods of reading and self testing are far better than marathon reading sessions followed by multiple mock exams.
- Self testing is the only way to assess what you know and what you don't know.
- Group revision can be very helpful for some and unhelpful for others. Find out early if this works for you or not. Any group revision session has to be structured and not just an opportunity to unwind or wind each other up!
- Do not panic if your revision is not going to plan. Find a mentor to help you get back on track.

- Remember that a 'healthy body equals a healthy mind'. Eat well and exercise to maintain energy levels and relieve stress. It is not healthy to shut yourself away for 3 months and it is not wise to tire yourself out by partying every weekend.

Points to remember

- Get an early night the day before so that you are fresh for the exam
- Arrive in good time and remember to bring all the documents requested
- Practice on the examination centre website beforehand to get a feel for using the system
- Manage your time carefully
- Read the questions carefully and select your answers carefully
- If you are unsure skip the question and you can go back to it afterwards
- Guess any questions at the end because there is no negative marking and so it is worth putting an answer down anyway
- Check for silly mistakes if you still have time
- Keep watching the clock (200 questions in 3 hours)

Single Best Answer (SBA) Question Paper

does this matter for ACEi/ARB

Cardiovascular problems – Hypertension

1. A 60 year old Afro-Caribbean male with known hypertension is already taking both amlodipine 10 mg and bendroflumethiazide 2.5 mg daily. His blood pressure still remains elevated at 165/105 mmHg.

    According to NICE hypertension guidelines, which is the **SINGLE MOST** appropriate next step in management? Select **ONE** option only.

    A. Add in a beta-blocker
    B. Add in an alpha-blocker
    C. Add in furosemide
    D. Add in ramipril
    E. Add in an angiotensin-II receptor antagonist

Cardiovascular problems – Heart Failure

2. According to NICE guidelines, choose from the following list of beta-blockers the only one that is licensed for use in heart failure. Select **ONE** option only.

    A. Atenolol
    B. Bisoprolol — *also carvedilol*
    C. Propranolol
    D. Metoprolol
    E. Sotalol

Cardiovascular problems – Secondary Prevention of Myocardial Infarction

3. A 58 year old man has been recently discharged from hospital following a myocardial infarction.

   Which of the following medications is **NOT** considered as essential secondary prevention to reduce mortality? Select **ONE** option only.

   A. Aspirin
   B. Amlodipine ——
   C. Simvastatin
   D. Ramipril
   E. Atenolol

Cardiovascular problems – Atrial Fibrillation

4. Which of the following is **NOT** a cause of atrial fibrillation?

   Select **ONE** option only.

   A. Hypothyroidism *hyper!*
   B. Mitral stenosis
   C. Ischaemic heart disease
   D. Caffeine
   E. Haemochromatosis ——

   may be caused by any condition causing atrial dilatation

Metabolic problems – Lipid Management *– go over*

5. A 49 year old man has a fasting lipid profile checked as part of his annual occupational health check-up. Taking his smoking status and blood pressure into account, his 10 year risk of cardiovascular disease is calculated to be 28%. After full discussion, he decides to start simvastatin 40 mg at night.

   What should his target cholesterol level be in accordance with NICE guidance? Select **ONE** option only.

   A. Total cholesterol <4 mmol/L
   B. Total cholesterol <5 mmol/L
   C. Total cholesterol:HDL ratio of <4.5
   D. Total cholesterol: HDL ratio of <5.5
   E. A target cholesterol level is not appropriate in this case

Cardiovascular problems – Atrial Fibrillation

6. A 45 year old man sees you with a 36 hour history of palpitations. There is no associated chest pain or shortness of breath and he has no past medical history of note. Cardiovascular examination is normal, apart from a fast irregular pulse. Electrocardiogram confirms atrial fibrillation with a rate of 120 beats per minute only.

   Which is the **SINGLE MOST** appropriate next step of management. Select **ONE** option only.

   A. Add aspirin + beta-blocker
   B. Add aspirin + warfarin
   C. Add digoxin + aspirin
   D. Add digoxin + warfarin
   E. Admit patient to hospital

Cardiovascular problems – Heart Failure

7. An 80 year old man has known chronic heart failure secondary to left ventricular systolic dysfunction. He is already on aspirin, simvastatin, bisoprolol, furosemide and ramipril. He says he is still getting short of breath on minimal exertion (e.g. walking 20 metres). On examination, his chest sounds clear and he has minimal pedal oedema.

   Which is the **SINGLE MOST** appropriate next step of management. Select **ONE** option only.

   A. Change bisoprolol to atenolol
   B. Refer to cardiologist
   C. Stop aspirin
   D. Add angiotensin-II receptor antagonist
   E. Add spironolactone

Neurological problems – TIA / Stroke

8. For a person who has had an ischaemic stroke or a TIA, what is the recommended NICE guidance to prevent further vascular occlusive events?

    Which is the **SINGLE MOST** appropriate option from the list below. Select **ONE** option only.

    A. Start clopidogrel
    B. Lifelong aspirin and take dipyridamole modified-release for 1 year only
    C. Lifelong aspirin and take dipyridamole modified-release for 2 years only
    D. Take both aspirin and dipyridamole modified-release lifelong
    E. Initiate warfarin therapy

Neurological problems – Dementia

9. According to NICE guidance, which of the following standard instruments should **NOT** be used in formal cognitive testing to help diagnose dementia?

    Select **ONE** option only.

    A. Mini Mental State Examination (MMSE)
    B. 7-minute screen
    C. General Practitioner Assessment of Cognition (GPCOG)
    D. Mental Aptitude Test (MAT)
    E. 6-Item Cognitive Impairment Test (6-CIT)

Neurological problems – Alzheimer's disease

10. Which of the following, according to NICE guidance, should **NOT** be used for cognitive symptoms and maintenance of function in Alzheimer's disease?

    Select **ONE** option only.

    A. Donepezil
    B. Aripiprazole
    C. Galantamine
    D. Rivastigmine
    E. Memantine

Neurological problems – Transient Ischaemic attack

11. An 82 year old woman with known hypertension comes to see you for review. Yesterday, she had a 3 hour episode of weakness in both her left arm and left leg. This is her first ever episode and there were no associated symptoms. Neurological examination is normal when she sees you. Her blood pressure is 160/105 and her only regular medication is bendroflumethiazide.

    Which is the **SINGLE MOST** appropriate next step in management. Select **ONE** option only.

    A. Start aspirin 300 mg od + specialist review within 24 hours
    B. Start aspirin 300 mg od + specialist review within 1 week
    C. Start aspirin 300 mg od + specialist review within 2 weeks
    D. Specialist review within 24 hours
    E. Start aspirin 75 mg od + request outpatient CT brain scan

Care of older adults – Falls

12. According to NICE guidance of assessment and prevention of falls, which of the following is **NOT** part of a multifactorial falls assessment?

    Select **ONE** option only.

    A. Identification of falls history
    B. Assessment of urinary incontinence
    C. Assessment of cognitive impairment and neurological examination
    D. Cardiovascular examination and medication review.
    E. Assessment of hearing

Care of people with learning difficulties – Autism

13. Which of the following is **NOT** associated with autism?

    Select **ONE** option only.

    A. Self-harm
    B. Hallucinations and delusions
    C. Few friends of the same age
    D. Repetitive behaviours
    E. Poor verbal communication is usually not supported with non-verbal communication

Genetics in primary care – Trisomy 21

14. A patient has Trisomy 21. Which of the following features is **NOT** associated with this condition?

Select **ONE** option only.

A. Epicanthic folds on lateral aspects of eyes.
B. Mental retardation
C. Alzheimer's disease
D. Transverse tongue fissures
E. Brushfield spots on the iris

Skin problems – Rash

15. A 40 year old man presents with a very itchy, widespread, papular rash for the last few days. His partner also has a similar rash. He has not used anything new recently. On examination, he has papules all over his body including his penis. A few odd burrows can be seen in his finger-web spaces.

Which is the **SINGLE MOST** appropriate next step of management? Select **ONE** option only.

A. Treat with oral antihistamines for 1 week and review if no better
B. Patient should apply permethrin 5% cream
C. Patient and any close contacts should apply permethrin 5% cream
D. Prescribe hydrocortisone 1% cream to apply to papules twice daily for 1 week
E. Suggest the patient should also get tested for syphilis and HIV

Skin problems – Impetigo

16. Which of the following statements is **TRUE** about impetigo?

Select **ONE** option only.

A. It is caused by *Staphylococcus aureus*
B. Oral flucloxacillin is the treatment of choice
C. It is not very contagious
D. It is sexually transmitted
E. It is caused by *Candida albicans*

Skin problems – Atopic eczema in children

17. According to NICE guidance on atopic eczema in children, which of the following statements is **NOT** an indication for referral to dermatology?

Select **ONE** option only.

A. If you suspect eczema herpeticum
B. Atopic eczema is severe and has not responded to 1 week of topical therapy
C. The diagnosis is uncertain
D. If you suspect contact allergic dermatitis
E. All children with atopic eczema should be referred to dermatology

Skin problems – Itchy feet

18. A 17 year old boy who plays lots of football and athletics at school complains of an itchy rash on both feet for the last one week. On examination, he has flaking and maceration in the toe web spaces of both feet and on the borders of his feet.

Which is the **SINGLE MOST** likely diagnosis? Select **ONE** option only.

A. Eczema
B. Psoriasis
C. Tinea pedis
D. Tinea manuum
E. Tinea unguium

Digestive problems – Irritable Bowel Syndrome (IBS)

19. Which one of the following treatments have NICE guidelines said should **NOT** be recommended for somebody with Irritable Bowel Syndrome?

Select **ONE** option only.

A. Sterculia
B. Lactulose
C. Ispaghula husk
D. Methylcellulose
E. Senna

Digestive problems – Chronic diarrhoea

20. A 24 year old man presents with a 6 month history of diarrhoea and weight loss. He has also noticed an itchy rash has developed on his elbows recently.

Which is the **SINGLE MOST** appropriate next step in management? Select **ONE** option only.

A. Refer for colonoscopy
B. Refer for upper GI endoscopy and duodenal biopsies
C. Check anti-tissue transglutaminase (tTG) antibodies
D. Refer to a dermatologist
E. Tell patient to start a gluten-free diet immediately

Digestive problems – Epigastric mass

21. A 62 year old woman presents with a gradually worsening 'feeling of fullness' in the top part of her abdomen and loss of appetite for the last 6 months. She has also noticed that her trousers have become slightly looser around her waist recently. On examination, she has a large, firm, smooth epigastric mass and an enlarged, left supraclavicular lymph node.

Which is the **SINGLE MOST** appropriate next step of management. Select **ONE** option only.

A. Request routine abdominal ultrasound scan
B. Refer urgently to gastroenterologist under 14-day referral
C. Request urgent abdominal ultrasound scan
D. Refer routinely to a gastroenterologist
E. Trial of peppermint oil

Digestive problems – Inflammatory Bowel Disease

22. Which one of the following conditions is **NOT** associated with Inflammatory Bowel Disease?

Select **ONE** option only.

A. Aphthous ulcers
B. Pyoderma gangrenosum
C. Dermatitis herpetiformis
D. Erythema nodusum
E. Sacroiliitis

Digestive problems – Itchy bottom

23. A mother brings in her 4 year old son who complains of having an itchy bottom for the last week. The itchiness is worst at night. He is otherwise well in himself and examination of the perianal area reveals no abnormality.

    Which is the **SINGLE MOST** appropriate next step of management. Select **ONE** option only.

    A. Call the duty child protection officer
    B. Hygiene measures only
    C. Hygiene measures + single-dose mebendazole for patient
    D. Hygiene measures + single-dose mebendazole for the whole family
    E. Hygiene measures + single-dose mebendazole repeated after 2 weeks for the whole family

Digestive problems – Gastrointestinal symptoms

24. A patient presents with some gastrointestinal symptoms. Which one of the following symptoms from the history would be least consistent with a diagnosis of irritable bowel syndrome?

    Select **ONE** option only.

    A. Abdominal bloating
    B. 71 year old male
    C. Past medical history of migraines
    D. Passing mucous with stool
    E. Symptoms worse on eating

Digestive problems – Diarrhoea

25. A 22 year old final year medical student returned from her elective in Kenya a week ago. For the last week, she has had watery stools with lots of flatus and describes the diarrhoea as being 'explosive'. She has no fever, no vomiting, there is no blood in her stools and she is otherwise well. Stool culture is negative.

    Which is the **SINGLE MOST** appropriate next step of management. Select **ONE** option only.

    A. Repeat another stool culture before starting any treatment
    B. Trial of loperamide
    C. Treat with course of ciprofloxacin 500 mg bd for 7 days
    D. Treat with metronidazole 2 g daily for 3 days
    E. Treat with mebendazole 100 mg as a single dose

Information management and technology – NHS initiatives

26. Which of the following is **NOT** one of the National Health Service's initiatives in information management and technology?

    Select **ONE** option only.

    A. Choose and Book
    B. Book and Treat
    C. Electronic Care Record
    D. GP-to-GP records transfer
    E. Electronic prescribing

Information management and technology – Read Codes

27. NHS Coding for Health has brought in a new coding system to replace Read codes.

    What is the name of this new coding system? Select **ONE** option only.

    A. NHSRC
    B. DVOOD
    C. READIT
    D. SNOWMED CT
    E. SNOWFLAKE

Neurological problems – Tremor

28. A 68 year old man complains of finding it increasingly difficult to fasten the buttons on his shirts. His wife has noticed he is salivating and dribbling a lot and that his handwriting has become smaller. On examination, he has a resting tremor and his limbs have cog-wheel rigidity.

    Which is the **SINGLE MOST** appropriate next step in management? Select **ONE** option only.

    A. Trial of levodopa and see if symptoms improve
    B. Trial of selegiline
    C. Start a beta-blocker
    D. Refer to a neurologist
    E. Request a computerised tomography brain scan

Rheumatology/Musculoskeletal system – Chronic fatigue syndrome

29. Which of the following is **NOT** a feature of chronic fatigue syndrome (CFS)?

    Select **ONE** option only.

    A. Painful lymph nodes without pathological enlargement
    B. Post-exertional fatigue (usually delayed for 24 hours post-activity and slow recovery)
    C. Generalised muscle/joint pains without any evidence of inflammation
    D. Sore throat
    E. Symptoms must be present for at least 4 weeks for diagnosis of CFS

Neurological problems – Meningism

30. In suspected meningitis, one test of meningism is pain on straightening the knee when the hip is flexed.

    What is the name of this sign called? Select **ONE** option only.

    A. Brudzinski's sign
    B. Babinski's sign
    C. Kernig's sign
    D. Lhermitte's sign
    E. Uthoff's sign

Neurological problems – Peripheral nerve lesion

31. A 24 year old woman fell off her horse and landed on her left elbow. She now has clawing of her left ring and little fingers with numbness and tingling in these two fingers also.

    Which nerve correlates to these signs and symptoms? Select **ONE** option only.

    A. Radial nerve
    B. Median nerve
    C. Ulnar nerve
    D. Sciatic nerve
    E. Femoral nerve

Neurological problems – Paraesthesia

32. A 22 year old woman who is 6 months pregnant has recently noticed she been getting painful pins and needles in her right thumb, index and middle fingers and also in the lateral half of her ring finger. Symptoms are worst at night and relieved by shaking her arm.

Which nerve correlates to these signs and symptoms? Select **ONE** option only.

A. Median nerve
B. Ulnar nerve
C. Radial nerve
D. Sciatic nerve
E. Femoral nerve

Neurological problems – Peripheral nerve lesion

33. A 55 year old woman was recently diagnosed with a large, left-sided ovarian cancer which is not surgically treatable. She now finds it very difficult to bend her left knee. On examination, her left hamstrings are weak and she has a left foot-drop.

Which nerve correlates to these signs and symptoms? Select **ONE** option only.

A. Tibial nerve
B. Common peroneal nerve
C. Sciatic nerve
D. Femoral nerve
E. Ulnar nerve

Neurological problems – Peripheral nerve lesion

34. A 17 year old boy recently fractured his right tibia and fibula after being tackled during football. On examination, he has a right foot-drop and cannot evert his foot or extend the toes. He also has sensory loss over the dorsum of his foot.

    Which nerve correlates to these signs and symptoms? Select **ONE** option only.

    A. Tibial nerve
    B. Common peroneal nerve
    C. Sciatic nerve
    D. Femoral nerve
    E. Ulnar nerve

Rheumatology/Musculoskeletal system – Weakness

35. A 30 year old woman, with known hypothyroidism, presents with weakness in her upper arms for the last four months, especially when she brushes her long hair. She also complains of blurred vision which is worse towards the end of the day. On a recent visit to the optician she was told her vision was fine.

    Which is the **SINGLE MOST** likely diagnosis. Select **ONE** option only.

    A. Multiple sclerosis
    B. Myaesthenia gravis
    C. Chronic fatigue syndrome
    D. Polymyalgia rheumatica
    E. Polymyositis

Neurological problems – Seizure

36. A 21 year old postman recently had his first ever seizure a month ago and is currently being investigated by the neurologists. He asks you how long it will be before he can drive again.

    Which is the **SINGLE MOST** appropriate answer. Select **ONE** option only.

    A. 18 months off driving since seizure, with medical review before restarting driving
    B. 12 months off driving since seizure, with medical review before restarting driving
    C. 24 months off driving since seizure, with medical review before restarting driving
    D. 12 months off driving since seizure, without medical review before restarting driving
    E. He can start driving immediately if his planned CT brain scan is reported as normal

Neurological problems – Bell's palsy

37. Which one of the following statements is **NOT** true about Bell's palsy?

    Select **ONE** answer only.

    A. Most cases of it are unilateral
    B. Most cases make a full recovery
    C. The forehead is typically spared
    D. The forehead is typically affected
    E. It is due to herpes zoster infection

Eye problems – Visual disturbance

38. A 55 year old woman experiences flashing lights in the peripheries of her vision (especially in dimly lit rooms) and also several moving black dots in her vision. She has also noticed increased cloudiness of her vision. There is no associated eye pain and she is normally short-sighted.

    What is the **SINGLE MOST** likely diagnosis? Select **ONE** option only.

    A. Acute glaucoma
    B. Migraines
    C. Retinal detachment
    D. Amaurosis fugax
    E. Cataracts

Eye problems – Squint

39. A 2 year old girl is brought to see you by her mother who has noticed that her daughter is looking 'cross-eyed'. This is confirmed by the corneal light reflection test.

    Which is the **SINGLE MOST** appropriate next step of management. Select **ONE** option only.

    A. Refer to optometrist for an eye-patch
    B. Refer to paediatric physiotherapist for exercises to strengthen eye muscles
    C. Advise that eye surgery is usually delayed until five years of age
    D. Advise the mother that the squint should eventually correct itself
    E. Refer to ophthalmologist

Eye problems – Raised Intra-ocular pressure

40. An 80 year old man, with known asthma, is found to have raised intra-ocular pressures at a recent optician check-up. You refer him to ophthalmology for further management.

    Which is the **SINGLE MOST** likely drug he will be started on from the list below. Select **ONE** option only.

    A. Timolol
    B. Latanoprost
    C. Pilocarpine
    D. Dorzolamide
    E. Brimonidine

Eye problems – Tunnel vision

41. A 33 year old man has noticed that his night-time vision is deteriorating and he is also complaining of worsening tunnel vision. He recalls that his grandfather had a similar 'eye condition'.

    Which is the **SINGLE MOST** likely diagnosis? Select **ONE** option only.

    A. Onchocerciasis
    B. Cataracts
    C. Retinoblastoma
    D. Myopia
    E. Retinitis pigmentosa

The General Practice consultation

42. Regarding your consultation which of the following statements is **TRUE**?

    Select **ONE** option only.

    A. If you are naturally an introvert then trying to create 'false rapport' with patients is useless
    B. Doctors can learn to be more empathetic
    C. The most important factor affecting compliance is the patient's perception that 'doctor knows best'
    D. The conscious mind can think about more than thirty different topics during the consultation
    E. The traditional medical model is usually learnt once you start working as a doctor

The General Practice consultation

43. Regarding the use of the telephone either during your consultation with a patient or to carry out a consultation, which of the following statements is **NOT** true?

    Select **ONE** option only.

    A. Telephones can be used when speaking to a patient whose first language is not English such as the service Language Line
    B. Minor ailments and self limiting diseases are two situations for a telephone consultation
    C. Using the telephone during a consultation with a patient can be a distraction and affect the patient/doctor relationship
    D. If during a telephone consultation you realise that you need to examine the patient you can tell him to ring back if he becomes worried about his symptoms
    E. Telephone consultations can sometimes result in high call charges to patients

The General Practice consultation

44. Which of these actions are **NOT** part of the 'social skills model'?

    Select **ONE** option only.

    A. Your clinic runs on time
    B. You end up treating patients for more than one problem
    C. You tell your patient that they can call the out of hours doctors if their symptoms get worse
    D. Your patient accepts shared responsibility for their care
    E. You give the correct antibiotics for an infection

The General Practice consultation – Models

45. Which of these 'consultation models' is more a philosophy than a model?

    Select **ONE** option below.

    A. Berne (1964)
    B. Stott and Davis (1979)
    C. Byrne and Long (1976)
    D. Heron (1975, 1989)
    E. Balint (1957)

Patient safety – Risk management

46. Which of the actions below is **NOT** an element of an appropriate infrastructure for risk management?

    Select **ONE** option only.

    A. Putting the names and GMC numbers of doctors in public display in GP waiting rooms.
    B. Training all staff members regularly
    C. Developing a work-based culture that is open
    D. The creation of protocols that deal with specific incidents
    E. Sign posting avenues of support for patients and staff

Patient safety – Drug reporting

47. Which of the statements is **NOT** true regarding the reporting of an adverse effect of a medication?

    Select **ONE** option only.

    A. It should be documented in the patient's notes
    B. It should be reported to the Medicine and Healthcare products Regulatory Agency (MHRA).
    C. It should be reported using the yellow card system
    D. It should be reported to the Local Medical Committee (LMC)
    E. It could be used as a Significant Event Analysis (SEA)

Promoting equality and valuing diversity

48. One of the senior receptionists at your practice has informed you that she is 14 weeks pregnant. She has worked at your practice for just under 28 weeks. With regard to the following below please select the statement that is **NOT** true.

Select **ONE** option only.

A. She is entitled to 52 weeks maternity leave of which 39 weeks are paid maternity leave

B. If her income is higher than the fixed minimum she can claim Statutory Maternity Pay

C. Maternity leave can start at a maximum of 11 weeks prior to the woman's expected delivery date

D. The employee can return to work one week after delivery; provided her GP signs her off maternity leave

E. An employer can insist that maternity leave start 4 weeks prior to her due date if the employee takes a single day of sick leave due to a pregnancy related illness

Promoting equality and valuing diversity

49. A formerly male salaried GP in the practice has just undergone a gender re-assignment operation. She now wants to be known as Jayne. Which of these statements is **NOT** true?

Select **ONE** option only.

A. It would be unlawful to not renew her contract as the practice already had two female GPs.

B. When signing letters and prescriptions she would have to use her original name as stated on her first GMC certificate.

C. She should be permitted to use the female toilet

D. She will still need a chaperone when performing intimate examinations of women.

E. The practice has a legal responsibility to demonstrate how they are preventing the discrimination of transgender and homosexual doctors.

Healthy people: Promoting health and preventing disease

50. Which of these statements concerning the Wilson-Junger Criteria is **NOT** true?

    Select **ONE** option only.

    A. The cost of screening must be acceptable
    B. Facilities for post test counselling must be available
    C. Effective treatment must be available
    D. The population must accept the tests
    E. There must be effective treatment for localised disease

Healthy people: Promoting health and preventing disease

51. Regarding colorectal cancer which of these statements is **TRUE**?

    Select **ONE** option only.

    A. The majority of colorectal cancers have an hereditary cause
    B. Less than 40% of colorectal cancers are within reach of a digital rectal examination
    C. Faecal occult blood screening does not reduce mortality
    D. More than 80% of colorectal cancers are missed by faecal occult blood screening
    E. Sigmoidoscopy is an effective screening tool for up to 5 years

Care of children and young people

52. Which of these does **NOT** need an urgent or immediate paediatric surgical referral?

    Select **ONE** option only.

    A. A 6 week old baby who is vomiting after feeds has become projectile
    B. A 3 year old boy whose mother has just noticed that his foreskin is non-retractable
    C. A 4 year old who has refused to finish her dinner, complains of abdominal pain and has vomited once
    D. A 6 month old baby boy with colic and a few flecks of what looks like red current jam in his nappy
    E. A 15 day old baby who is exclusively breast fed and has jaundice and pale stools

Care of children and young people – Neonatal Jaundice

53. Regarding Jaundice in the neonate, which of these statements is **TRUE**?

    Select **ONE** option only.

    A. Jaundice within the first 24 hours is ALWAYS abnormal
    B. Jaundice is usually an indication to stop breast feeding
    C. Phototherapy must only be considered if there are contraindications to an exchange transfusion
    D. The presence of gut flora increases the retention of bile salts
    E. Prolonged jaundice occurs if it does not begin to fade within 14 weeks

Care of children and young people – Breast feeding

54. Which of the following statements concerning breast feeding/milk is **NOT** true?

    Select **ONE** option only.

    A. Breast milk contains lymphocytes
    B. Breast feeding protects against atopic eczema
    C. Breast milk reduces the risk of fatal hypernatraemia due to dehydration
    D. Breast milk reduces the risk of gastrointestinal infection in infants
    E. Breast milk has a greater concentration of iron than formula milk.

Care of children and young people – Disorders of Puberty

55. You see a mother who presents with her 7 year old girl who has begun to develop some alarming symptoms such as body odour. On examination you observe that she is tall for her age, has pubic and auxillary hair. Which of the following differential diagnoses is **LEAST** likely?

    Select **ONE** option only.

    A. Congenital Adrenal Hyperplasia
    B. A virilising ovarian tumour
    C. Maternal Diethylstilbestrol
    D. Cushing syndrome
    E. Polycystic ovarian syndrome

Care of acutely ill people

56. With regards to a possible diagnosis of meningococcal disease which of these symptoms/signs is **MOST** worrying?

    Select **ONE** option only.

    A. Cold extremities
    B. Neck pain
    C. A fine pink rash that blanches with pressure
    D. Mild headache, worsened by light but no papilloedema
    E. Symptoms lasting more than one week

Care of acutely ill people

57. A 21 year old female basketball player collapses after a training session. She is initially treated for exhaustion by the team doctor after having just returned from a tournament in the Far East. However, when she begins to develop shortness of breath and chest pain she is rushed to hospital. She does not take oral contraception nor does she smoke. Her initial X-ray is normal and her D-dimer is only mildly raised.

Which is the **SINGLE MOST** likely diagnosis. Select **ONE** option only.

A. Atypical Pneumonia
B. Hypertrophic Obstructive Cardiomyopathy (HOCM)
C. Pneumothorax
D. Pulmonary Embolism
E. Diaphragmatic irritation secondary to a ruptured ectopic pregnancy

Genetics in primary care

58. A couple visit you following the results of the heel prick test of their newborn baby son. He has been diagnosed with cystic fibrosis and they have been told that it was an autonomic recessive disease. They have another son and one daughter and are worried about their other children.

Which is the **SINGLE MOST** appropriate response. Select **ONE** option only.

A. The chance of the baby's siblings being affected is reduced as they have not yet been diagnosed
B. If the cystic fibrosis gene was inherited in an autonomic recessive manner than there is a 2/4 chance that his brother will be affected
C. The chances of both the baby and his brother having cystic fibrosis is 1/16
D. There is a theory that the disorder evolved as a mechanism of protection against malaria
E. The baby should be referred to a children's hospice

Care of people with cancer and palliative care

59. A 79 year old man with metastatic prostate disease presents in your clinic complaining of moderately severe back pain. He is already on hormonal treatment and takes only paracetamol for his pain.

    With regards to the WHO analgesic ladder which is the SINGLE MOST appropriate next step? Select **ONE** option only.

    A. Oromorph prn and a Fentanyl patch
    B. Ibuprofen tds
    C. TENS machine prn
    D. Codeine phosphate qds plus ibuprofen
    E. Morphine sulphate qds

Care of people with cancer and palliative care – Benefits

60. You see a 30 year old father of three who has just learnt that he has advanced bowel cancer. Amongst other worries he tells you that he has substantial financial worries as he is self employed.

    With regards to his terminal condition which of these statements concerning benefits is **TRUE**? Select **ONE** option only.

    A. He must have required help with normal functioning for at least one year to be eligible
    B. His savings must be below the maximum amount to be eligible
    C. He may be able to go on holiday with the aid of a charitable grant
    D. Only patients with a prognosis of less than four weeks can have their claims 'fast tracked'
    E. He must submit his persona bank statements to be assessed for disability allowance

Metabolic problems – Thyroid eye disease

61. Regarding the treatment of thyroid eye disease, which of these statements is **NOT** true?

    Select **ONE** option only.

    A. Smoking Cessation
    B. Use of Eye lubricants
    C. Referral to specialist centres
    D. Avoid Propyluracil
    E. Correct Thyroid dysfunction

Metabolic problems – Diabetes research

62. The ADVANCE Trial is the largest study of diabetes treatments. The study showed that intensive blood glucose lowering using modified release Gliclazide protects against serious complications. With regards to this which of these statements is **NOT** true?

    Select **ONE** option only.

    A. Hypoglycaemic attacks are reduced by 32%
    B. HbA1C is safely controlled at 6.5%
    C. Renal disease is reduced by 21%
    D. The risk of death due to cardiovascular is reduced but this is not statistically significant
    E. The development of macroalbuminuria is reduced by 30%

Metabolic problems – Diabetes

63. Regarding the future of anti-diabetic therapy which of the following is **NOT** presently available?

    Select **ONE** option only.

    A. Incretin mimetics
    B. Inhaled insulin
    C. Oral insulin
    D. Oral DPP-4 inhibitors
    E. Continuous subcutaneous insulin infusion (CSII)

Metabolic problems – Osteoporosis

64. You see a 75 year old woman who has just been discharged from hospital following a fracture of her wrist. With regards to the treatment of osteoporosis recommended by NICE which one of these statements is **TRUE**?

    Select **ONE** option only.

    A. You should refer her for an urgent DEXA scan
    B. You should treat her if she has a bone mineral density of less than –3 SD.
    C. You should treat her if her bone mineral density is less than 2.5 and she has a BMI of less than 19 kg/m^2.
    D. She is too old for a DEXA scan
    E. Teriparatide should be prescribed as the new first line agent

Respiratory problems – Asthma

65. You see a 3 year old girl who is having breathing problems due to her asthma despite treatment with her Salbutamol inhaler plus spacer. What is the next step in her management?

    Select **ONE** option only.

    A. Inhaled Beclomethasone 200–400 micrograms/day
    B. Long Acting Beta Antagonist
    C. Prednisolone 40mg
    D. Refer to a paediatrician
    E. Ipratropium Bromide

Respiratory problems – cough and night sweats

66. A 31 year old Jamaican man presented to your clinic 2 weeks ago with shortness of breath, wheeze, cough and night sweats. You sent him for an x-ray. The x-ray report mentions bilateral hilar enlargement. On further examination of the patient you discover non-tender ulcers on the backs of his arms and scalp.

    Which is the **SINGLE MOST** likely diagnosis? Select **ONE** option only.

    A. HIV
    B. Sarcoidosis
    C. Tuberculosis
    D. Non-Hodgkin's Lymphoma
    E. Systemic Lupus Erythematosus

Respiratory problems – Sinusitis

67. A 25 year old patient presents requesting antibiotics for his sinusitis. He has had symptoms for a week and does not believe it is just a common cold. Which one of these symptoms does **NOT** make sinusitis more likely than a simple upper respiratory tract infection?

    Select **ONE** option only.

    A. Nasal obstruction
    B. Tooth pain
    C. Pain when bending
    D. Unilateral maxillary pain
    E. Purulent rhinorrhoea

Metabolic problems – Metabolic syndrome

68. A 25 year old woman comes to you seeking advice on how to lose weight. On questioning she discloses that she was once told that she had metabolic syndrome. Which of these symptoms is **NOT** part of the diagnostic criteria for metabolic syndrome?

Select **ONE** option only.

A. Raised fasting glucose >5.6 mmol/L
B. Raised triglycerides >1.7 mmol/L
C. Reduced thyroxine > 8 pmol/L
D. Reduced high density lipoproteins
E. Raised blood pressure

Metabolic problems – Obesity

69. A 40 year old businessman with problems controlling his weight requests an 'anti-obesity' tablet. He does not fit the criteria to be prescribed any weight loss medication. He says that he will buy some over the counter anyway. Which of these drugs is available without a prescription?

Select **ONE** option only.

A. Orlistat
B. Sibutramine
C. Rimonabant
D. Metformin
E. Exenatide

Men's health – Prostate problems

70. Which of the following symptoms is **NOT** part of the International Prostate Symptom Score?

Select **ONE** option only.

A. Increased frequency
B. Increased urgency
C. Nocturia
D. Dysuria
E. Straining

Rheumatology/Musculoskeletal system – Foot problems

71. A 50 year old overweight woman presents with pain in her right heel. She reports it is worst first thing in the morning when she gets up. On examination she has pain on palpation of the inferior aspect of the heel.

    Which is the **SINGLE MOST** likely diagnosis. Select **ONE** option only.

    A. Gout
    B. Osteoarthritis
    C. Achilles tendonitis
    D. Plantar fasciitis
    E. Pes planus

Metabolic problems – Eating disorders

72. Which of the following is **NOT** a feature of anorexia nervosa except?

    Select **ONE** option only.

    A. Low FSH
    B. Low LH
    C. High cortisol
    D. High growth hormone
    E. High potassium

Sexual health – Vaginal discharge

73. A 25 year old woman presents with an offensive, fishy smelling vaginal discharge. She says it is watery in nature.

    Which is the **SINGLE MOST** likely diagnosis. Select **ONE** option only.

    A. Bacterial vaginosis
    B. Candida
    C. Chlamydia
    D. Trichomonas
    E. Gonorrhoea

Sexual health – Methods of contraception

74. A 38 year old woman wants to have a copper IUD fitted. She has asked how long it will take for it to become effective?

Select **ONE** option only.

A. 7 days
B. 5 days
C. 2 days
D. Immediately
E. 14 days

Women's health – Endometriosis

75. Which of the following is **NOT** a common symptom of endometriosis?

Select **ONE** option only.

A. Pelvic pain
B. Dyspareunia
C. Dysmenorrhoea
D. Dysuria
E. Vaginal bleeding

Women's health – Antenatal care

76. According to the NICE 2008 Antenatal care guidelines, which of the following is **TRUE**?

Select **ONE** option only.

A. Women should have routine auscultation of the foetal heart
B. Women should have routine screening for Chlamydia
C. On each antenatal visit they should have a pelvic examination
D. In an uncomplicated pregnancy for a nulliparous women she should have 7 appointments
E. Screening for sickle cell disease should be offered to all women

Sexual health – Combined oral contraceptive

77. A 17 year old girl comes to see you in the family planning clinic. She is taking Microgynon 30 tablets. She normally remembers to take her pills on time everyday but she forgot to take one of her pills yesterday and she had unprotected sexual intercourse last night. It has been less than 24 hours since she missed the pill and she is 2 days into her current pack.

    Which is the **SINGLE MOST** appropriate management option? Select ONE option only.

    A. Emergency contraception needed
    B. Perform a pregnancy test
    C. Take missed pill immediately and continue packet as normal
    D. Advise use of condoms for the next 7 days
    E. None of the above

Research and academic activity – Screening tests

78. When comparing the specificity of two different screening tests what type of significance test should be used?

    Select **ONE** option only.

    A. Spearman's rank
    B. Chi squared
    C. Pearson's test
    D. Wilcoxon matched pairs
    E. Student's t-test

Men's health – Drug side effects

79. Which of the following is **NOT** a side effect of finasteride when used for benign prostatic hypertrophy?

    Select **ONE** option only.

    A. Erectile dysfunction
    B. Loss of libido
    C. Gynaecomastia
    D. Ejaculation problems
    E. Dizziness

Rheumatology/Musculoskeletal system – Joint problems

80. A 50 year old known alcoholic develops pain and swelling of his right metatarsophalangeal joint.

    Which is the **SINGLE MOST** likely diagnosis. Select **ONE** option only.

    A. Gout
    B. Pseudogout
    C. Psoriatic arthritis
    D. Septic arthritis
    E. Trauma

Personal and professional responsibilities – Employment rules

81. An employee must be provided with a written contract of employment by the employer within how long after starting a new job?

    Select **ONE** option only.

    A. 2 weeks
    B. 2 months
    C. 3 months
    D. 4 weeks
    E. 3 weeks

Care of people with mental health problems – Management of depression

82. According to NICE guidelines which one of the following is recommended for cognitive behavioural therapy for depression?

    Select **ONE** option only.

    A. Fear fighter
    B. Beating the blues
    C. Overcoming depression
    D. COPE
    E. OC Fighter

Sexual health – Pelvic inflammatory disease

83. In Britain, which organism is the most common cause of Pelvic Inflammatory Disease?

Select **ONE** option only.

A. Trichomonas vaginalis
B. Neisseria gonorrhoea
C. Candida
D. Chlamydia trachomatis
E. Bacterial vaginosis

ENT and facial problems – Laryngitis

84. Which one of the following is a predisposing factor for developing laryngitis?

Select **ONE** option only.

A. Under use of voice
B. Alcohol
C. Diet
D. Not smoking
E. Drugs

Metabolic problems – Osteoporosis

85. Which one of the following is **NOT** a risk factor for developing osteoporosis?

Select **ONE** option only.

A. Immobility
B. Family history
C. Long term steroid use
D. Late menopause
E. Asian origin

Healthy people: promoting health and preventing disease – Smoking cessation

86. Which of the following is **NOT** a common side effect of varenicline?

Select **ONE** option only.

A. Nausea
B. Headache
C. Abnormal dreams
D. Insomnia
E. Menorrhagia

Sexual health – Human Papilloma virus vaccine

87. Which of the following regarding the Human Papilloma Vaccine is **NOT** true?

Select **ONE** option only.

A. Cervarix is given in 3 stages
B. Cervarix protects against HPV 6, 11, 16 and 18
C. HPV is the main aetiological factor in developing cervical cancer
D. It is effective if given before sexual activity starts
E. An alternative vaccine is called Gardasil

Clinical governance – Quality Outcome Framework

88. Out of all the available QOF points, how many are available for clinical domains?

Select **ONE** option only.

A. 757
B. 44
C. 167.5
D. 91.5
E. 1060

Patient safety – Notifiable diseases

89. Which of the following is **NOT** a notifiable disease?

Select **ONE** option only.

A. TB
B. Measles
C. Mumps
D. Herpes zoster
E. Tetanus

Clinical ethics and values based practice – Prescription charges

90. For which of the following conditions do patients still have to pay for prescriptions?

Select **ONE** option only.

A. Diabetic on insulin
B. Hypothyroidism
C. Hyperthyroidism
D. Epileptic on medication
E. Hypoparathyroidism

Sexual health – Combined pill

91. Which of the following statements about the combined contraceptive pill is **NOT** true?

Select **ONE** option only.

A. Protects against cervical cancer
B. Protects against endometrial cancer
C. Protects against ectopic pregnancy
D. Reduces number of functional ovarian cysts
E. Increases the incidence of breast cancer

Women's health – Breast cancer

92. Which of the following factors does **NOT** increase the risk of breast cancer?

Select **ONE** option only.

  A. Late menarche
  B. Late menopause
  C. Family history of breast cancer
  D. Increasing age
  E. Combined oral contraceptive

Women's health – Pre-eclampsia

93. At how many weeks gestation can pre-eclampsia be labelled?

Select **ONE** option only.

  A. 24 weeks
  B. 28 weeks
  C. 32 weeks
  D. 20 weeks
  E. 12 weeks

Women's health – Menopause

94. Menopause is defined as how many months of spontaneous amenorrhoea?

Select **ONE** option only.

  A. 6 months
  B. 24 months
  C. 12 months
  D. 18 months
  E. None of the above

Care of people with mental health problems

95. A 48 year old woman presents with multiple physical symptoms for which investigations and reviews have revealed no organic cause. What is this an example of?

    Select **ONE** option only.

    A. Panic disorder
    B. Somatisation disorder
    C. Munchausen's syndrome
    D. Conversion disorder
    E. Hypochondrial disorder

Care of people with mental health problems – Switching between anti-depressants

96. A patient taking citalopram for her depression has had no real improvement after 3 months. The GP has decided to start her on venlafaxine. How is the anti-depressant meant to be switched?

    Which is the **SINGLE MOST** appropriate response. Select **ONE** option only.

    A. Stop the citalopram straight away and then start the venlafaxine
    B. Withdraw the citalopram and then start the venlafaxine the next day
    C. Cross taper the withdrawal of citalopram with the commencement of venlafaxine
    D. Wait 2 weeks after stopping the citalopram before starting the venlafaxine
    E. None of the above

Care of people with mental health problems – Treatment of schizophrenia

97. According to the NICE guidelines on schizophrenia, what is the treatment of choice for newly diagnosed schizophrenia?

Select **ONE** option only.

A. Lithium
B. Clozapine
C. Haloperidol
D. Olanzapine
E. Sertraline

ENT and facial problems – Centor criteria

98. Which one of the following is **NOT** part of the Centor criteria?

Select **ONE** option only.

A. Absence of a cough
B. History of a fever
C. Pain on swallowing
D. Tender anterior cervical lymphadenopathy
E. Presence of a tonsillar exudate

Rheumatology/Musculoskeletal system – Back pain

99. Which of the following is a treatment recommended according to the recent NICE guidelines on management of non-specific low back pain?

Select **ONE** option only.

A. TENS
B. Acupuncture
C. Injection into back
D. SSRIs
E. Laser therapy

Rheumatology/Musculoskeletal system – Rheumatoid arthritis

100. Which of the following statements is **NOT** true according to the NICE guidelines on Rheumatoid arthritis?

Select **ONE** option only.

A. Refer patient urgently if there has been delay of 2 months or longer between development of symptoms and seeking help

B. In newly diagnosed active RA, offer a combination of disease modifying anti-rheumatic drugs, including methotrexate and at least one other, plus a short term glucocorticoid.

C. CRP and key components of disease activity should be monitored monthly until disease is controlled

D. If NSAIDs are prescribed they should be at the lowest effective dose for the shortest time possible

E. Patients should have access to a named member of the MDT responsible for co-ordinating their care.

Answer Section: Single Best Answer

1. D
    See NICE guidance (2006) – if patient is already on a calcium-channel blocker and thiazide diuretic, then the next step is to add an ACE-inhibitor.

    For more information see the NICE quick reference guide at http://www.nice.org.uk/nicemedia/pdf/cg034quickrefguide.pdf

2. B
    NICE guidance on chronic heart failure (2003) recommended bisoprolol and carvedilol were the only beta-blockers that should be licensed for use in heart failure.

    For more information see the NICE guideline guide at http://www.nice.org.uk/nicemedia/pdf/CG5NICEguideline.pdf

3. B
    NICE guidance (2007) says that calcium channel antagonists should not routinely be used for secondary prevention.

    For more information see the NICE quick reference guide at http://www.nice.org.uk/nicemedia/pdf/CG48QuickRefGuide.pdf

4. A
    Hyperthyroidism and thyrotoxicosis are usually associated with atrial fibrillation (AF). Any condition that causes dilatation of the atria will cause AF.

5. E
    Primary prevention – simvastatin 40 mg (or equivalent) should be offered to adults over 40 with a 10-year cardiovascular disease risk of >20%. There is no target total cholesterol or LDL cholesterol for 1° prevention.

Secondary prevention – all patients with clinical evidence of CVD should be on simvastatin 40 mg (or equivalent) unless contraindicated. Simvastatin should be increased to 80 mg if total cholesterol does not drop to <4mmol/L or LDL cholesterol does not drop to <2 mmol/L.

For more information see the NICE quick reference guide at http://www.nice.org.uk/nicemedia/pdf/CG67quickrefguide.pdf

6. E

For AF with onset < 48 hours, you should admit the patient for heparinisation, followed by a trans-thoracic echocardiogram (to exclude a thrombus). If no thrombus, patient can either have DC cardioversion or pharmacotherapy, (amiodarone if structural heart disease or flecainide if no structural heart disease).

For AF with onset > 48 hours, the patient needs therapeutic anticoagulation for at least 3 weeks. If there is high risk of cardioversion failure (e.g. previous failure or recurrent AF), then the patient needs at least 4 weeks of amiodarone or sotalol prior to DC cardioversion.

After DC cardioversion, they need anticoagulation for at least 4 weeks, after which a decision needs to be made about further anticoagulation, based on individual case risk assessment.

For more information see the NICE quick reference guide at http://www.nice.org.uk/nicemedia/pdf/CG036quickrefguide.pdf

7. E

NICE guidance recommends adding spironolactone at this stage.

For more information see the NICE guideline at http://www.nice.org.uk/nicemedia/pdf/CG5NICEguideline.pdf

8. C

NICE guidance (2005) states that for people who have had a transient ischaemic attack/stroke (ischaemic) – they should take aspirin and dipyridamole MR for 2 years. Thereafter, or if dypridamole MR not tolerated, preventative therapy should revert to standard care (including prophylaxis with low-dose aspirin).

For more information see the NICE quick reference guide at http://www.nice.org.uk/nicemedia/pdf/TA090quickrefguide.pdf

9. D

    NICE guidance on dementia (2006) states that MMSE, 7-minute screen, GPCOG and 6-CIT should be used in helping to diagnose dementia.

    For more information see the NICE quick reference guide at http://www.nice.org.uk/nicemedia/pdf/CG042quickrefguide.pdf

10. B

    Acetylcholinesterase inhibitors (especially donepezil) are the mainstay of treatment in Alzheimer's disease (AD). NICE guidance on dementia (2006) suggests donepezil, galantamine and rivastigmine can all be used for moderately severe AD (MMSE 10-20 points). Memantine (NMDA-receptor antagonist) is only recommended for mild AD. Aripiprazole is an anti-psychotic licensed for use in schizophrenia.

11. A

    See NICE guidance on stroke/TIA (2008). Here is the ABCD2 prognostic scoring system for suspected transient ischaemic attack:

	Criteria	Points
A	**A**ge = 60 years	1
B	**B**lood pressure = 140/90	1
C	**C**linical features: – Unilateral weakness – Speech disturbance, no weakness	2
D	**D**uration of symptoms: – > 60 mins – 10 – 59 mins	2 1
	Diabetic	1

If a person's ABCD2 score is ≥4, then they need aspirin 300mg daily and specialist review within 24 hours. The same applies if they have crescendo transient ischaemic attacks (≥2 per week).

For more information see the NICE guidance at http://www.nice.org.uk/nicemedia/pdf/CG68QuickRefGuide.pdf and http://www.nice.org.uk/nicemedia/pdf/TA090quickrefguide.pdf

12. E

For more information see the NICE quick reference guide at http://www.nice.org.uk/nicemedia/pdf/CG021quickrefguide.pdf

13. B

Autism is characteristically associated with a triad of impairments in social interaction, imaginative thought and communication. Symptoms usually present before the age of three years old.

14. A

Epicanthic folds are on their medial aspects of eyes.

15. C

These symptoms suggest Scabies. Scabies is due to mite Sarcoptes scabei infestation. Spread is mainly via skin-to-skin contact and through infested clothing. Also sexually transmitted. Common spread in households and institutions (e.g. nursing homes). First-line treatment is permethrin 5% cream and second-line is malathion 0.5% liquid. Patients and close contacts must be treated at the same time.

16. A

Impetigo is a superficial skin infection due to either *Staphylococcal aureus* or *Streptococcus pyogenes.* It is highly contagious and therefore children must be kept away from school until all lesions have crusted or healed. Treatment is with topical fucidic acid or mupirocin (or oral flucloxacillin if widespread).

17. E

For further information see NICE guidance at, http://www.nice.org.uk/nicemedia/pdf/CG057QuickRefGuide.pdf

18. C

Tinea pedis is the commonest dermatophyte infection and it occurs on the feet, mostly in the toe spaces, but can also spread to the soles, heels and borders of the foot. It is common in adolescents and young adults. Treatment is with topical antifungal creams (e.g. miconazole cream twice daily for 4 weeks).

Tinea manuum is a dermatophyte infection of the hand. Tinea unguium is a dermatophyte infection of the nail.

19. B

NICE guidance (2006) states that laxatives should be considered in the management of Irritable Bowel Syndrome, but not lactulose.

20. C
NICE guidelines (2009) recommend that testing for Coeliac disease (serological and intestinal biopsy) is only accurate if patient is following a gluten-containing diet. Patients are not to start a gluten-free diet until Coeliac disease has been confirmed by a gastroenterologist on intestinal biopsy (even if serological tests are positive).

For more information see the NICE quick reference guide at http://www.nice.org.uk/nicemedia/pdf/CG86QuickRefGuide.pdf

21. B
NICE guidance on referral for suspected cancer (2005) suggests that urgent referral is required for any patient with an upper abdominal mass, even if it is without dyspepsia.

For more information see the NICE quick reference guide at http://www.nice.org.uk/nicemedia/pdf/CG027quickrefguide.pdf

22. C
Dermatitis herpetiformis is usually associated with Coeliac disease. It is an intensely itchy vesicular rash, which is symmetrical and commonly found on the extensor surfaces (elbows, knees, buttocks, back and back of the neck).

23. D
Threadworm (Enterobius vermicularis) infestation is quite common. An itchy bottom without any other concerns does not warrant referral to child protection team.

Threadworm infestation may present as perianal itching which is worst at night, and girls may have vulval symptoms. It can be diagnosed by putting sellotape around the anus and sending it to the laboratory for microscopy to see the eggs. However, this is not necessary and empirical treatment can be given.

The Clinical Knowledge Summary guidelines recommend hygiene measures + an antihelminthic for all members of the household. Mebendazole is used first-line for children >6 months old and only a single dose is given, unless infestation persists.

For more information see the clinical knowledge summaries website at http://www.cks.nhs.uk/threadworm/management/quick_answers#-262926

24. B

See recent NICE guidelines (2008) on diagnosis and management of Irritable Bowel Syndrome (IBS). In this, onset of symptoms in someone over 60 years old is considered a red flag. Past history of migraines has no bearing on a diagnosis of IBS.

For more information see the NICE guidance at http://www.nice.org.uk/nicemedia/pdf/CG61IBSQRG.pdf

25. D

Giardiasis is the most likely culprit. It is due to the flagellate protozoan Giardia lamblia and presents as outlined in the case. Its incubation period is 2 weeks. If suspected, treat empirically with metronidazole. Rapid response is diagnostic.

26. B

Choose & Book – allows patients to choose which hospital/clinic they wish to go to in order to see a specialist (once their GP feels a specialist referral is warranted). Patients can also choose the date and time of their appointment.

Electronic Care Record – basic data about patients is made available online, so care in situations such as emergencies can be given quicker and safer.

GP-to-GP records transfer – patient records can be transferred electronically between GP surgeries.

Electronic prescribing – GPs and practice nurses can send prescriptions electronically to whichever pharmacy a patient wishes.

27. D

SNOWMED CT: Systematized Nomenclature of Medicine – Clinical Terms. It will be used as the new standard terminology for the NHS Care Records Service by NHS 'Connecting For Health'.

28. D

Parkinson's disease (PD) should be suspected in anyone with symptoms of tremor, stiffness, slowness, balance problems +/– gait problems. NICE guidelines (2006) state that patients with suspected PD should be referred untreated to a neurologist for assessment and diagnosis.

For more information see the NICE quick reference guide at http://www.nice.org.uk/nicemedia/pdf/cg035quickrefguide.pdf

29. E

Chronic fatigue syndrome is associated with post-exertional fatigue or malaise, chronic pain, sleep disturbance, cognitive difficulties (see NICE guidance for full list of symptoms – need to be present for at least 4 months).

For more information see the NICE quick reference guide at, http://www.nice.org.uk/nicemedia/pdf/CG53QuickRefGuide.pdf

30. C

This is Kernig's sign. Brudzinski's sign is involuntary lifting of the legs when the neck is flexed in meningism. Babinski's sign is a plantar extensor response which can indicate upper motor neurone damage in adults. Lhermitte's sign – in multiple sclerosis, you get a sensation of 'electric shocks' running down the spine when neck is flexed. Uthoff's sign is where multiple sclerosis symptoms worsen in response to heat (e.g. hot bath) or to exercise.

31. C

She has damaged her ulnar nerve at the elbow.

32. A

This is median nerve compression or carpal tunnel syndrome. It is associated with pregnancy, rheumatoid arthritis, hypothyroidism and trauma. Night-time symptoms can be managed with a wrist-splint, but severe symptoms may need surgery to decompress the median nerve in the carpal tunnel.

33. C

She has a sciatic nerve mononeuropathy due to compression from her pelvic tumour. Other causes of sciatic neuropathy include back pain.

34. B

This is common peroneal nerve damage which is most commonly due to trauma.

35. B

Myaesthenia gravis is an autoimmune disorder which presents as weakness of the periocular, shoulder girdle, bulbar and facial muscles. It is due to antibodies which cause loss of muscle acetylcholine receptors. It is associated with rheumatoid arthritis, hypo/hyperthyroidism, polymyositis and systemic lupus erythematosus. Fifteen percent of cases will have thymoma.

36. B

See the DVLA's guidance for more information at http://www.dvla.gov.uk/medical/ataglance.aspx

37. C

Forehead is only spared in upper motor neurone lesions (due to bilateral innervations of frontalis muscle).

38. C

Retinal detachment presents as a painless loss of vision (like a 'shadow' or 'curtain' spreading across the field of vision. About 50% have preceding flashing lights or spots. Causes: idiopathic, diabetes (fibrous bands in vitreous humour), post-cataract surgery, myopia. This needs urgent ophthalmological referral to securely fix the retina back.

39. E

Squint (strabismus) is characterised by abnormal coordinated eye movements due to misalignment of the visual axes.

There are 2 main types: concomitant (common) and paralytic (rare)

Concomitant squint – due to imbalance in extraocular muscles (convergent more common)

Paralytic squint – due to paralysis of extraocular muscles

Tests:

(1) Cover light reflection test – hold pen-torch 30cm away from child's face and see if light reflects symmetrically on both pupils

(2) Cover test – ask child to focus on subject, cover one eye and observe movement in uncovered eye. Then cover other eye and repeat test.

All cases should be referred to the ophthalmologist to determine nature/severity of squint and to exclude serious causes. Eye-patching will help prevent amblyopia ('lazy eye').

40.   B
Prostaglandin analogues (e.g. latanoprost) are used as first line treatment in patients with asthma and they work by increasing uvoscleral flow.

Beta-blockers (e.g. timolol) decrease aqueous production, but should be avoided in patients with asthma and heart failure

Miotics (e.g. pilocarpine) decrease uvoscleral flow. Side effects include small pupil, headache and blurred vision

Sympathomimetics (e.g. brimonidine) decrease aqueous production and increase outflow. They should be avoided if taking MAOI's and tricyclic antidepressants.

Carbonic anhydrase inhibitors (e.g. dorzolamide) decrease aqueous production

41.   E
Retinitis pigmentosa is an inherited disorder leading to gradual deterioration of the light-sensitive cells of the retina. It usually presents with night-time blindness, tripping over things and deterioration of peripheral vision (central vision in some cases). Symptoms usually become noticeable between the ages of 10-40 years old.

42. B

Empathy can be learnt by recognising strong feelings in patients and trying to imagine how they might feel. It is important to try and create a rapport with patients even if this does not come naturally to you. Good communication skills come naturally to some lucky individuals but they can always be improved. Concordance is a better term than compliance and is achieved when an agreement is reached between a patient and their doctor regarding which treatment is the most efficient way of achieving the patient's goals. This must involve an exchange of information between the patient and their doctor so that each is better informed with regards to the disease and the patient's illness respectively (i.e. the illness being defined as the effect of the disease on the patient). The final therapeutic decision is a shared one that might be mutually agreed, negotiated or even one that splits opinion but in which the patient's beliefs and wishes are the main priority. The conscious mind can only think about a much smaller number of issues at one time and so it is important to communicate clearly with patients to retrieve the most important information. The traditional model of medicine has been taught in medical schools for many years whilst other more personalised models are usually learnt once a doctor has started seeing patients independently.

43. D

If a patient needs to be examined then you have to see them. For instance for a first episode of vertigo in a middle-aged smoker can you really be sure that this patient only has labrinythitis and not a cerebellar infarct? Companies that offer interpretation services make use of telecommunications and although not perfect using a telephone during the consultation is a more confidential way of consultation with a person whose first language is not English than by use of a friend or relative who speaks both languages. Minor self limiting illnesses often do not need a face to face consultation and time and money can be saved by consulting with these patients over the phone. Some practices use 084 numbers which put callers into a queue rather than making them listen to an engaged tone. However, these numbers are more expensive to call and if a patient has to wait a long time then these costs can build up.

44. C
Safety netting is part of Neighbour's checkpoints not Pendleton's doctor's tasks otherwise known as the social skills model

Pendleton *et al.* 1984/2003

i.   Define reason for patient's attendance
ii. Consider other problems
iii. Negotiate an appropriate action for each problem
iv. Achieve a shared understanding of the problem
v.   Involve the patient in the management and encourage them to accept appropriate responsibility.
vi. Use time and resources appropriately
vii. Establish and maintain a relationship with the patient

Neighbour 1987, 2004

i.   Connecting – establishing rapport with patient
ii. Summarizing – clarifying the reason for the consultation
iii. Handing over – negotiating and agreeing a management plan
iv. Safety netting – planning for the unexpected and managing uncertainty
v.   House keeping – the doctor is aware of their own emotions

45. E
Balint, 'The doctor, His patient and The Illness' is a philosophical publication that states that psychological problems are often manifest as physical symptoms; that doctors feelings have a role in the consultation and that doctors need to be trained to understand what is going on in the minds of their patient's during the consultation.

46. A
The names of doctors and GMC numbers are already published on the GMC website. The other answers help reduce or manage risk by giving them skills and instructions to deal with specific incidents. Therefore this reduces stress levels amongst staff and also avoids a blame culture following adverse incidents.

47. D

    The LMC are the BMA's representative in GP pay negotiations and represent local GPs in other areas. They also provide training and support to GPs and aim to improve communication in general practice. The patient should be informed of any adverse effect of a medication and this should be documented in their notes. The MHRA accept the yellow cards in the back of the BNF and use these to monitor the adverse incidents of drugs. A SEA can help prevent adverse incidents from recurring.

48. D

    A woman may return to work from maternity leave 2 weeks post partum or 4 weeks postpartum if she works in a factory. Of note is the fact that employers can force female employees to start their maternity leave early if they take a single day off work with a pregnancy related problem so classifying a patient's problem as pregnancy related can have financial and social consequences.

49. B

    Many female doctors change their maiden name to their married name with the GMC. Briefly look at these Acts; Sexual Discrimination Act 1986, Employment Equality Regulations 2003, Gender Recognition Act 2004. It is not acceptable to put a cap on the number of employees of a certain sex, race, sexuality or disability. Anyone who is classified a female under the law can use the female toilets and facilities. Chaperones are advised for intimate examinations regardless of the sex of the patient or doctor. All public bodies have a duty to positively promote equality and diversity.

50. B

    This is not part of the criteria. Other criteria include:

    - The condition must be important
    - There is a detectable early stage
    - The natural history of the disease is understood
    - Appropriate screening intervals are known
    - The psychological, physical and emotional risks are less than the perceived benefits.

51. B

However, it is still important to perform this examination on any patient for whom you suspect this diagnosis. 40% of colorectal cancers are missed by faecal occult blood screening but it does reduce mortality and a national screening programme has been recommended.

52. B

A = Congenital pyloric stenosis (occurs 6–8 weeks) and requires a pyloromyomectomy

B = Phimosis – it is usual up to the age of 4 years and a 'wait and see' approach is usual prior to perhaps starting Betamethasone cream

C = This could be appendicitis, although rare in under-fives it is associated with a 90% perforation rate in these patients.

D = Intussusception, occurs between 5 and 12 months and has a 3:1 male to female ratio

E = Congenital Biliary Atresia – suspect in any baby with prolonged jaundice (>14 days)

53. A

Jaundice is always abnormal within the first 24 hours and could be due to sepsis or haemolysis (ABO or Rhesus Incompatibility or a red cell abnormality). Physiological Jaundice occurs due to the ABSENCE of gut flora to eliminate bile salts, due to hepatic immaturity and reduced fluid intake due to breast feeding. It is not usually a reason to stop breast feeding.

54. E

Breast milk has less iron than formula milk but infants absorb a greater percentage of iron from breast milk than from formula milk. There is still a debate as to whether breast fed infants require supplemental iron. Breast milk also contains less sodium chloride and potassium than formula milk, so reducing the risk of hypernatraemia secondary to dehydration.

55. C

Diethylstilbestrol (DES) use during pregnancy increases the risk of breast cancer in female offspring and hypospadias in male offspring.

56. **A**

Cold extremities, leg pain and rapid progression are all red flag signs of meningococcal disease. Many viral infections can cause a non-specific rash. The ability to perform fundoscopy can help to (but not comprehensively) exclude photophobia.

57. **D**

She has a positive D-dimer. Despite there being only a small rise if you suspect the diagnosis enough to perform this test than you should act on the results. The D-dimer is just a marker aid to deciding how probable a PE is and does not provide a definitive answer.

58. **C**

¼ x ¼ = 1/16. Patients can be diagnosed later on in life and the odds are not changed by time of diagnosis. There is a hypothesis that it evolved as a mechanism of protecting people against cholera as the disease prevents the fatal salt losses associated with cholera diarrhoea. Sickle cell anaemia is thought to protect against malaria due to the inability of the vector to survive in the host's red blood cell.

59. **D**

Learn the WHO analgesic ladder i.e.

1. Pain: non-opioid +/– adjuvant
2. Mild-moderate pain despite previous drugs: weak opioid +/– non-opioid and/or adjuvant
3. Persistent pain despite previous analgesia: strong opioid +/– non-opioid and/or adjuvant.

60. **C**

In order to look after patients with a terminal illness you must treat them holistically. This includes directing them to areas of financial/ emotional or spiritual support. Good websites include the Douglas MacMillan and Cancer Research.

61. **D**

The treatment of thyroid eye disease is often under valued despite the fact that it can prevent blindness and social isolation. Read the article in the BMJ on thyroid eye disease (Perros. P. BMJ 2009;338:b560).

62. A

Hypoglycaemic attacks can occur with sulphonylureas as they promote insulin secretion. This is especially true in elderly patients. The ADVANCE trial has a website: www.advance-trial.com. This is worth a browse.

63. C

The insulin would become denatured in the stomach acid. Incretins are released by the intestines after eating and stimulate insulin secretion. Incretin mimetics are injected subcutanously 1 hour prior to the patient's morning and evening meals. They cause the secretion of insulin when required amongst other actions. DPP-4 is an enzyme that breaks down incretins.

64. D

You should treat any female patient over 75 with a fracture for osteoporosis without requesting a DEXA scan. Thus answers A, B and C are incorrect. Bisphosonates are first line medication for osteoporosis whereas Teriparatide is used only in patients who can not use bisphosphonates or strontium ranelate.

65. A

For more information see the SIGN guidance at h ttp://www.sign. ac.uk/pdf/qrg101.pdf

66. B

This is a condition that occurs more often in Afro-Caribbean families than people of European descent and also affects these people more severely.

67. A

Sinusitis is a common problem and you should be aware of the red flag signs of the condition. There is a good article in the InnovAiT journal (Jan 2009, Vol 2, Issue 1).

68. C

Metabolic syndrome is associated with cardiovascular disease, diabetes and gout.

69. A

Is now available OTC as Alli.

70. D

The International Prostate symptom score was developed and validated by the American Urological Association. It has seven questions each scored out of 5. The questions cover frequency, nocturia, weak urinary stream, hesitancy, incomplete emptying, urgency and intermittency. Dysuria is not a symptom of this scoring system.

71. D

Plantar fasciitis is a common cause of inferior heel pain caused by inflammation of the ligamentous insertion of plantar fasci into the calcaneum. Pain is usually worse first thing in the morning when taking the first few steps after getting out of bed. It is usually unilateral and settles within 6 weeks. Management is to advise on better footwear with good arch support, heel padding and soft heels, treatment with NSAIDs and steroid injections and structure-specific plantar fascia-stretching program or standard Achilles tendon-stretching protocol. The other options would not cause this presentation.

72. E

Anorexia nervosa is a psychophysiological condition, occurring especially in girls and young women characterised by the inability or refusal to eat. The prevalence rate of this condition is estimated at 1 to 2% of schoolgirls and female students in higher education. It affects men much less. Onset in females is usually between the ages of 16 and 17 years and it unusual for it to start after the age of 30. The main clinical features of the condition are a reduced body weight, with a body mass index < 17.5, an intense desire to remain thin and amenorrhoea in females. Physical problems include dry skin, lanugo hair, hypothermia, hypotension, sensitivity to the cold, hypokalaemia not hyperkalaemia. Treatment is mainly with psychological treatment. Bulimia nervosa is another eating disorder. This is more common than anorexia nervosa. In bulimia nervosa there is binge eating with feelings of guilt or loss of control. It is not usually associated with weight loss. Treatment is with psychological intervention using an evidence based self-help programme but also treatment with anti-depressants of which fluoxetine is recommended.

For more information see www.gpnotebook.co.uk and NICE guidance at http://www.nice.org.uk/nicemedia/pdf/cg009quickrefguide.pdf

73. A

The answer is bacterial vaginosis. The Amsel criteria are used to diagnose this and you need 3 of the following:

- thin, white homogeneous discharge
- clue cells on microscopy of wet mount
- pH of vaginal fluid >4.5
- release of a fishy odour on adding alkali

For more information on this see www.bashh.org

74. D

Copper IUDs are effective immediately. They are an example of a long-acting reversible contraceptive (LARC). They work by preventing fertilisation and inhibiting implantation. With 380 mm^2 copper they can be licensed for 5–10 years. If a woman is 40 or older when it is inserted it can be kept in until she no longer needs contraception. If pregnancy does occur the risk of ectopic is 1 in 20, the risk of uterine perforation is 1 in 1000. It can make periods heavier.

For more information see the NICE quick reference guide at http://www.nice.org.uk/nicemedia/pdf/cg030quickrefguide.pdf

75. D

Endometriosis is a common disorder in which there are endometrial glands and stroma outside of the endometrial cavity. It affects about 15% of women. It is most commonly found in the pelvis but can be anywhere. It is a benign condition. It is more common in women 30–40 and Caucasians. It regresses during pregnancy and after the menopause (if not on oestrogen replacement). Combined oral contraceptive users have a lower incidence. Risk factors are family history, heavy periods and frequent cycles. The aetiology is not known but there are several theories such as retrograde menstruation and metaplasia of coelomic derivatives. It presents with pelvic pain, dyspareunia, dysmenorrhoea, menorrhagia and infertility. Dysuria is not a common symptom. Investigation is with laparoscopy and transvaginal ultrasound. The extent of endometriosis found on laparoscopy does not correlate with the severity of symptoms. If there is pelvic pain treatment is with pain relief and hormonal treatment. Referral may be needed and surgery required. Infertility also needs referral.

76. E

Screening for sickle cell disease should be offered to all women. In an uncomplicated pregnancy for a nulliparous woman she should have 10 appointments- parous women should have 7 appointments. Routine auscultation of the foetal heart and routine pelvic examination is NOT recommended. Women do NOT need routine screening for Chlamydia.

For more information see the NICE quick reference guide at http://www.nice.org.uk/nicemedia/pdf/CG062QuickRefGuide.pdf

77. C

When taking Microgynon 30mcg pills, if one or two are missed, then the woman should take the missed pill as soon as she remembers and then take pills as normal. No additional contraceptive protection is needed.

If 3 or more pills are missed, then she should take the missed pill as soon as possible and then take pills as normal. She should use condoms or abstain from sex until 7 pills have been taken in a row.

If the missed pills are in week one of her cycle then emergency contraception is needed if the woman had sex during her pill free interval or in week one of her cycle.

If the pills were missed in week 2 of her cycle, there is no need for emergency contraception as she would have had 7 pills in a row already.

If the pills were missed in week 3 of her cycle then she should finish the current pack and omit the pill free interval.

For more information see the Faculty of Sexual and Reproductive Healthcare guidance at www.ffprhc.org.uk/admin/uploads/MissedPillRules%20.pdf

78. B

Chi squared should be used when comparing two different tests. Chi squared is a test used for non-parametric date (which is not normally distributed). Other tests for non-parametric data include Mann-Whitney, Wilcoxon and Spearman's rank. Parametric data is normally distributed and tests for this include; the Student t-test and Pearson's. Make sure you know about the various statistical tests and terms.

79.   E
Benign prostatic hyperplasia is a common condition in older men. It is unusual before 50 years of age and is most common between 60 and 70. Many patients are asymptomatic or have mild disease. Only 20% of those over 60 years have disease sufficiently severe to warrant surgery. Patients present with obstructive symptoms such as terminal dribbling, double micturition, hesitancy and straining. It also presents with irritative symptoms such as nocturia, urgency, frequency. In those with mild or moderate symptoms watchful waiting is an option. If symptoms are troublesome then medical treatment with an alpha blocker such as doxazosin can be used. Side effects of this include dizziness and postural hypotension. Another drug that can be used is finasteride which is a 5-alpha reductase inhibitor. Side effects of this are loss of libido, gynaecomastia, ejaculation problems and erectile problems. This takes up to 6 months to work. Surgery is left for severe symptoms.

For more information see www.gpnotebook.co.uk

80.   A
Gout is a disorder of purine metabolism in which you get acute, recurrent attacks of synovitis due to urate crystal deposition. It is more common in men and increases with age. Predisposing factors are a family history, high alcohol intake, high purine diet, diuretics, infection, surgery, obesity, cytotoxics and renal failure. Patients present with a painful, hot, swollen joint (most commonly big toe, ankles, fingers). Serum urate may be raised and aspiration and polarised light examination shows negatively birefringent crystals. Treatment is with rest, increased fluid intake, NSAIDs (colchicine as an alternative). For prophylaxis allopurinol and uricosuric drugs are used.

81.   B
Rules about employment and staff issues are very important within General Practice. The employer must give (and have signed by both parties) the written contract within 2 months. See www.direct.gov.uk for more information.

82. B

This is the recommended choice by NICE for mild and moderate depression. Fear fighter is recommended for people with panic and phobia. There is not enough evidence to recommend COPE or Overcoming depression. OC fighter is for obsessive-compulsive disorder.

For more information see the NICE guidance at http://www.nice. org.uk/nicemedia/pdf/TA097guidance.pdf

83. D

Pelvic inflammatory disease is a spectrum of inflammatory conditions affecting the upper genital tract with Chlamydia accounting for at least 50%. Chlamydia and gonorrhoea can co-exist. It is a major cause of infertility and ectopic pregnancy. Risk factors include age 15–24, sexual activity, IUD, previous PID, surgical procedures such as termination of pregnancy and tubal surgery. Symptoms include lower abdominal pain, vaginal discharge, fever, vomiting, dysuria, dyspareunia and menstrual irregularities. Some women are asymptomatic and it is found on investigation for infertility. On examination there may be cervical excitation and adnexal tenderness. Treatment is with ofloxacin 400 mg bd and metronidazole 400 mg bd for 2 weeks. Contact tracing through the GUM should be carried out.

For more information see www.gpnotebook.co.uk

84. B

Laryngitis is inflammation of the larynx or vocal cords. It is usually caused by a virus and is self limiting but can be bacterial. Symptoms include hoarseness, malaise and fever or pain on using voice. Predisposing factors include alcohol, smoking and overuse of the voice. Treatment is with rest, analgesia, antibiotics if bacterial infection and steam inhalation.

85. D

Other risk factors include rheumatoid arthritis, high alcohol intake, long term steroid use, previous fracture, parental history of a hip fracture.

86.   E
Varenicline (Champix) is a partial agonist at the nicotine receptor. It alleviates the symptoms of craving and withdrawal. Treatment with this should start 1–2 weeks before the target stop date. It may be associated with nausea and vomiting, headache, drowsiness, gastro-intestinal disturbances. Menorrhagia is a less common side effect. The usual course of treatment is 12 weeks.

For more information see the NICE guidance at http://www.nice. org.uk/nicemedia/pdf/TA123Guidance.pdf

87.   B
Gardasil protects against these 4. Cervarix protects only against 16 and 18. They are both given as IM injections as 3 doses at intervals 0, 1 and 6 months. The target age group are girls of 12–13 years old.

88.   A
This is the number of points available for clinical domains which include CHD, Stroke and TIA, Left Ventricular dysfunction, AF, Hypertension, Hypothyroidism, CKD, DM, Obesity, Mental Health, Learning disability, Depression, Dementia, COPD, Asthma, Epilepsy, Cancer, Palliative care and Smoking. The other areas are organisational domains, holistic care, patient experience and additional services. For more information see Quality Outcomes Framework guidance for GMS contract 2009/10 document at www. bma.org.uk/images/qof0309_tcm41-184025.pdf

89.   D
Certain diseases are required to be notified to the consultant responsible for Communicable Disease Control under the Public Health (Control of Disease) Act 1984. Diseases include: Acute encephalitis, Anthrax, Cholera, Diptheria, Food poisoning, Malaria, Measles, Meningitis, Mumps, Rubella, Scarlet fever, Tetanus, Tuberculosis, Typhoid fever, Viral hepatitis, Whooping cough, Yellow fever.

90.   C
It is underactive hormone conditions which allow exemption from paying. These include Diabetes (unless diet controlled), Hypoadrenalism, Hypopituitarism, Myaesthenia gravis, Epilepsy needing continuous anti-convulsants, Myxoedema/requirement for thyroxine or hypoparathyroidism.

91. A

All the other statements are true. The combined pill decreases the risk of ovarian and endometrial cancer but increases the risk for cervical cancer and breast cancer.

92. A

It is early menarche that is a risk factor and not late menarche.

93. D

Pre-eclampsia affects 5–7% of primigravida and 2–3% of all pregnancies. It occurs in the second half of pregnancy after 20 weeks gestation and resolves usually within 10 days after delivery. It is characterised by pregnancy induced hypertension with proteinuria and often oedema. The cause is not known and once present it does not improve until the baby has been delivered. Women are also at greater risk of getting hypertension later on.

Risk factors include previous pre-eclampsia, family history of pre-eclampsia, age ≥40, nulliparity, pregnant with a new partner, interval of more than 10 years between pregnancies, multiple pregnancy, BMI ≥35, renal disease or vascular disease. Smoking is not a risk factor. Symptoms include headache, oedema of face, hands or feet, vomiting, abdominal pain, visual problems such as flashing or blurring.

The British Hypertension Society uses the following criteria to diagnose pre-eclampsia – rise of diastolic blood pressure ≥15mmHg or systolic ≥30mmHg above booking blood pressure OR diastolic blood pressure ≥90 mmHg on 2 occasions 4 hours apart or diastolic ≥110 mmHg on 1 occasion and proteinuria (> 0.3 g/24 hr). Management of pre-eclampsia is to deliver the baby.

For more information see www.gpnotebook.co.uk

94. C

Menopause is the cessation of periods. It occurs in the UK on average at 51 years old. It is defined as 12 months amenorrhoea with no other cause in women. There is an increase in FSH and LH as the negative feedback from oestrogen diminishes. Symptoms include vasomotor symptoms such as hot flushes and night sweats, urogenital symptoms such as vaginal dryness, atrophy and urinary incontinence, psychological problems such as low mood and anxiety. It also increases the risk of IHD and osteoporosis. Hormone replacement is the main treatment.

95. B
Somatisation disorder is when a patient has multiple physical symptoms present for at least 2 years and the patient refuses to accept negative test results or reassurance.

96. B
SSRIs are the recommended anti-depressant initially as they are as effective as tricyclics but less likely to be discontinued due to side effects. If there has been no response after a month you can consider switching to a different anti-depressant. When switching from an SSRI to venlafaxine you should withdraw the SSRI, start venlafaxine the next day (37.5 mg/day) and increase very slowly. The exception to this is fluoxetine. With fluoxetine you should wait 4–7 days until venlafaxine is started as fluoxetine has a long half-life and active metabolites.

For more information see the Clinical Knowledge Summaries website at http://cks.library.nhs.uk/home

97. D
Schizophrenia is a condition in which there is disturbance in the form and content of thought. There is a lifetime prevalence of 1% and it has a peak age of onset of 15–25 years old for men and 25–35 years old for women. Schneider's first rank symptoms include – auditory hallucination (hearing thoughts spoken out loud, hearing voices referring to them in third person or running commentary), thought withdrawal, insertion or removal, thought broadcasting, somatic hallucinations, delusional perception, feelings or actions experienced as made or influenced by external agents. For newly diagnosed schizophrenia first line treatment is with atypical anti-psychotics, such as olanzapine.

98. C
Centor criteria are absence of cough, history of fever, presence of tonsillar exudates and tender anterior cervical lymphadenopathy or lymphadenitis. Pain on swallowing is not part of the centor criteria. If three or more of the criteria are present then immediate antibiotic prescribing should be considered for acute tonsillitis/ acute pharyngitis/sore throat.

For more information see the NICE guidance at http://www.nice.org.uk/nicemedia/pdf/CG69QRG.pdf

99. B

The others are options that are not meant to be offered for management. Other recommended options include manual therapy and structured exercise programmes.

For more information see the NICE quick reference guide at http://www.nice.org.uk/nicemedia/pdf/CG88QuickRefGuide.pdf

100. A

Rheumatoid arthritis is the most common disorder of connective tissue affecting about 1% of the population. It affects women about 2–4 times more than men. It can occur at any age. It is multifactorial but there is a large genetic component. It usually starts with symmetrical small joint involvement. All patients with suspected rheumatoid arthritis should be referred to rheumatology. It can have both articular and extra-articular manifestations. X-ray may show loss of joint space, erosions and joint destruction. Rheumatoid factor is positive in the majority of patients. Patients should be referred if there has been a delay of 3 months or longer between development of symptoms and seeking help.

For more information see the NICE guidance at http://www.nice.org.uk/nicemedia/pdf/CG79QRGv2.pdf

Extended Match Question (EMQ) Paper

Digestive problems – Vitamin deficiency

A. Vitamin A
B. Vitamin C
C. Vitamin D
D. Vitamin E
E. Vitamin K
F. Thiamine
G. Niacin
H. Vitamin B6
I. Vitamin B12
J. Folic acid

For each of the features below, select the **SINGLE MOST** appropriate vitamin deficiency from the options above. Each option may be used once, more than once or not at all.

1. Dermatitis, dementia and diarrhoea
2. Bleeding gums and teeth
3. Glossitis, confusion and peripheral neuropathy
4. Neural tube defects
5. Night blindness

Evidence-based practice – Alternative medicine

A. Benign prostatic hypertrophy
B. Common cold
C. Migraines
D. Depression
E. Hot flushes
F. Irritable bowel syndrome
G. Osteoarthritis
H. Asthma

For each of the following herbal medicines below select the **SINGLE MOST** appropriate medical condition that it is most associated with from the above options. Each option may be used once, more than once or not at all.

6. Peppermint oil
7. Saw Palmetto — BPH
8. St John's Wort
9. Feverfew — migraines
10. Echinacea — common cold

Women's health – Breast disorders

A. Fibroadenoma
B. Fibroadenosis
C. Breast cancer
D. Lipoma
E. Mammary duct ectasia
F. Breast abscess
G. Fat necrosis
H. Paget's disease of the breast
I. Sebaceous cyst

For each of the following cases below select the **SINGLE MOST** appropriate diagnosis from the options above. Each option may be used once, more than once or not at all.

11. A 25 year old woman who comes to see her GP with a non-tender, mobile lump felt within her right breast.

12. A 50 year old woman who has found a hard, tender, irregular lump in her breast. There is a history of breast cancer within her family.

13. An obese woman who has had a fall recently presents with a hard, irregular breast lump.

14. A 29 year old woman who is currently breast feeding presents with a tender, red and hot left breast.

15. A 53 year old woman comes to see you and mentions she is suffering from a green discharge from her right nipple and also feels a tender lump near this area.

Women's health – Pregnancy

A. Inevitable miscarriage
B. Threatened miscarriage
C. Incomplete miscarriage
D. Missed miscarriage
E. Recurrent miscarriage
F. Normal pregnancy
G. Ectopic pregnancy
H. Still birth

For each of the cases below select the **SINGLE MOST** appropriate diagnosis from the options above. Each option may be used once, more than once or not at all.

16. A pregnant woman at 8 weeks gestation presents with vaginal bleeding. On examination the cervical os is closed and an intrauterine pregnancy is seen on the ultrasound scan.

17. A woman who is 10 weeks pregnant presents with abdominal pain and vaginal bleeding and pain and on examination her cervical os is open and she has passed large clots.

18. A woman gives birth to a baby at 25 weeks gestation that is dead.

19. A woman has her booking ultrasound scan and this shows no foetal pole.

20. A woman has abdominal pain and vaginal bleeding. On examination she has cervical excitation and her last period was nine weeks ago.

Personal and professional responsibilities – Sick Notes

A. Med 3
B. Med 4
C. Med 5
D. Med 6
E. SC 1
F. SC 2
G. RM7
H. DS 1500

For each of the cases below select the **SINGLE MOST** appropriate note from the options above. Each option may be used once, more than once or not at all.

21. Used when it is thought to be harmful to put the actual diagnosis on the sick note
22. Used when patient is undergoing the Personal Capability Assessment
23. Self-certification form used when person is eligible to claim statutory sick pay
24. A man comes to see you in the practice and wants a sick note from work. On examination you find he has mechanical back pain and feel he needs a few weeks off work.
25. The form requested by a patient with a terminal illness as they want to speed up the process of receiving their attendance allowance.

Rheumatology/Musculoskeletal system – Back pain

A. Paget's disease
B. Rheumatoid arthritis
C. Osteoarthritis
D. Ankylosing spondylitis
E. Multiple myeloma
F. Disc prolapsed
G. Mechanical back pain
H. Malignancy

For each of the cases below select the **SINGLE MOST** appropriate diagnosis from the options above. Each option may be used once, more than once or not at all.

26. A 40 year old complains of sudden onset of severe back pain radiating down to the right foot

27. A 65 year old man has progressive back pain. His blood tests show renal failure and a high ESR.

28. A 20 year old man presents with early morning back pain and stiffness and he has a high ESR.

29. An elderly woman with pain on movement in her right knee. It settles with rest.

30. 70 year old man has had a 7 month history of weight loss and back pain. He has also had increasing urinary frequency.

Men's health – Urological problems

A. Testicular torsion
B. Epididymitis
C. Testicular cancer
D. Prostate cancer
E. Benign prostatic hypertrophy
F. UTI
G. Prostatitis

For each of the cases below select the **SINGLE MOST** appropriate diagnosis from the options below. Each option can be used once, more than once or not at all.

31. A 54 year old man with a PSA of 7ng/dl and an enlarged prostate on examination
32. A 70 year old man with lower urinary tract symptoms, an enlarged prostate on examination and a PSA of 3ng/dl
33. A young boy who develops pain and swelling of his left testicle. There is no relief on lifting the testicle up.
34. A man who is 35 years old notices a lump in his right testicle.
35. A man who has been having dysuria and has a positive urine dipstick for nitrites and leucocytes

Rheumatology/Musculoskeletal system – Joint and bone problems

A. Septic arthritis
B. Osteoarthritis
C. Rheumatoid arthritis
D. Osteoporosis
E. Gout
F. Pseudogout
G. Psoriatic arthritis
H. Osteopaenia

For each of the cases below select the **SINGLE MOST** appropriate diagnosis from the options below. Each option may be used once, more than once or not at all.

36. An elderly woman with pain in her right knee which is worse on exertion, also with joint space narrowing on her x-ray
37. A 68 year old woman with a DEXA scan t score more than 2.5 standard deviations below the mean
38. A 62 year old woman with a DEXA scan t score of 1.5 standard deviations below the mean.
39. A 24 year old man presents with a painful right knee. On examination it is red, hot, tender and swollen. He is not able to move the knee.
40. A 56 year old woman presents with distal interphalangeal joint swelling and pain as well as nail dystrophy.

The General Practice Consultation – Theoretical models

A. The medical model (1971)
B. Balint (1957)
C. Berne (1964)
D. The Health Belief Model (1966)
E. Byrne and Long (1976)
F. Stott and Davis (1979)
G. Helman (1981, 2007)
H. Heron (1975, 1989)
I.   Pendleton et al (1984, 2003)
J. Neighbour (1987, 2004)
K. Kurtz and Silverman (1996, 2002)

For each example below, select the **SINGLE MOST** appropriate consultation model from the options above. Each option can be used once, more than once or not at all.

41. A 40 year old woman has come to see you for a routine blood pressure check. As you ask her about her attempts to modify her lifestyle she begins to giggle and answers your questions in a childish manner. You try to find out why her attempts at smoking cessation have failed but find that by the end of the consultation you feel like you have had to chastise her.

42. You have just broken bad news to a patient. During the consultation he wanted to know what had happened to him; why he had contracted the disease; why had it only begun to affect him now; what would happen if he just ignored the disease: how would it affect his wife; what he should do: and who should he turn to for more information

43. Your Clinical Supervisor would like you to demonstrate a consultation model whilst he observes you. He particularly wants you to define the reason for the patient's attendance plus any other problems they might want to share, achieve a shared understanding of the patient's problems and create a management plan that is appropriate, where responsibility is shared between yourself and the patient. He also wants you to use your time and the practice resources appropriately whilst establishing a relationship with the patient.

44. You see a patient who regularly attends your practice asking for sick notes despite the fact that you believe he is fit enough to return to work. You decide to confront him with your belief.

45.   You see an anxious mother near the end of a busy Friday afternoon clinic. Her child has a low grade pyrexia, otalgia and mild headache. You diagnose otitis media, prescribe Amoxicillin and advise the mother to bring the child to the out-of-hours doctor or A+E if her symptoms get worse, if she develops photophobia or neck stiffness. You have 5 more patients to see but decide to have a cup of coffee as you are exhausted.

Patient safety

A. Use NPSA Incident Decision Tree
B. Perform Significant Event Analysis
C. Improve Staff training
D. Be open and fair
E. Use yellow card system
F. Report to MHRA
G. Inform Child Protection Officer
H. Perform an Audit
I. Complete Multi-Source Feedback
J. Inform the police
K. Report to the GMC or NMC

For each example below, select the **SINGLE MOST** appropriate option above. Each option can be used once, more than once or not at all.

46. You are a GP principal in a large practice. A patient has just successfully sued the practice for an adverse incident related to an erroneous prescription. You want to know the root cause of the mistake.

47. An 18 month old girl has had a reaction to a newly licensed medication you prescribed on the previous consultation. You suspect that it is due to an interaction with an over the counter medication the mother has given to the child but neglected to tell you when you prescribed the medication. You want to stop this from happening again.

48. As a GP trainee you are shocked to see the foundation one doctor in your practice shouting at a patient. This isn't the first time you have seen her behave this way. You ask her about this and she tells you not to worry as the patient is a bit stupid and won't follow her instructions properly. You offer to help her improve her communication skills but she tells you she has very good communication skills.

49. A receptionist at your practice has recently left having given poor advice to a patient who called the practice complaining of chest pain and later died of a myocardial infarction. The other reception staff, think that she has been made a scapegoat as the practice nurse had also been present when the phone call was received. As GP principal you are under pressure from the Primary Care Trust to act.

50. You see a 75 year old man with palpitations and a past medical history of heart failure and chronic kidney disease. You notice that although he is on Spironolactone he has not had his urea and electrolytes checked in over a year.

Promoting equality and valuing diversity

A. Race Relations Amendment Act (2000)
B. Race Relations Act (1976)
C. Equal Opportunities Commission
D. Sexual Discrimination Act (1975, 1986)
E. Commission for racial Equality/Equality and Human Rights Commision
F. Employment Equality Regulations (2003, 2003, 2006)
G. Disability Discrimination Act (2005)
H. Maternity and parental leave etc. and the paternity and adoptive leave(amendment) regulations (2006)
I. Building Act (1984)
J. Mental Health Act (1983, 2007)
K. Children's Act (1989, 2004)

For each example below, select the **SINGLE MOST** appropriate option from the above list. Each option can be used once, more than once or not at all.

51. A homosexual male GP has been refused 2 weeks paid leave to spend with the baby he's adopted with his partner. Which regulation has not been followed?

52. You are one of three GP partners at a struggling rural practice. At a practice meeting the practice manager tells you that she thinks that a ramp needs to be fitted at the practice entrance and that this must be paid for from the practice budget. Your partners dispute this but she says that there is legal responsibility on the practice to allow disabled patients to come to the surgery.

53. A salaried GP who graduated in Iraq has not has his contract renewed as the GP principle is worried about the plight of recently qualified British GPs and wants to employ a British GP. The salaried GP takes his case to an industrial tribunal.

54. A recently qualified female GP has been unsuccessful in a job interview. During the interview she was asked about how her children felt about her working hours, if she intended to extend her family, whether she had previously had time off due to "women's problems" or to look after her children. She believes that her interviewer was wrong to ask these questions as she thinks her children benefit from having a doctor as a mother. She wants to make a complaint about the practice.

55. A practice manager is advertising for a new receptionist. She creates a job application form in which there are questions about race. The practice nurse questions whether she is allowed to include this question and if the practice needs a policy to prevent racial discrimination but the practice manager ignores her concerns as the practice had never been accused of racism in the past. The practice nurse finds information on the internet that describes the responsibility of the practice to promote equality and diversity.

Care of children and young people – Developmental milestones

A. 22 months
B. 4 months
C. 8 years
D. 6 years
E. 2 and 1/2 years
F. 10 Months
G. 5 months
H. 10 weeks
I. 4 years
J. From birth
K. 13 months

For each example below, select the **SINGLE MOST** appropriate developmental age from the options above. Each option can be used once, more than once or not at all.

56. Knows two words other than 'mama' and 'dada'.
57. Draws a man and includes six parts of the body
58. Grasps rattle
59. Builds a tower of four cubes
60. Gives first and last name

Genetics in Primary Care

A. X-linked recessive
B. Autosomal Dominant
C. Trisomy 21
D. Robertsonian Translocation
E. Triplet repeat (Anticipation)
F. Incomplete Penetrance
G. Autosomal recessive
H. Trisomy 13
I.   X linked Dominant
J. Klinefelter's Syndrome
K. Imprinting

For each example below, select the **SINGLE MOST** appropriate genetic term which is being described from the options above. Each option can be used once, more than once or not at all.

61. You see a male patient whose son has Down's syndrome. He has been told by a geneticist that any future offspring will have a greater than 50% chance of having the disorder.

62. A mother of a girl with severe learning difficulties, epilepsy, ataxic gait and a generally happy disposition has been researching her daughter's condition on the internet. She is distressed to have learnt that the causative genetic abnormality could only have come from her and not her husband.

63. You see an 18 year old man who tells you that he is increasingly worried about his prognosis. His Grandfather had Huntington's disease and managed to cope with the symptoms for many years. His father inherited the disease but his symptoms were much worse and he has recently committed suicide.

64. You see a female patient who is recovering from a still birth. On post mortem the foetus had severe cardiac malformations and bilateral cleft lip and palate.

65. A young mixed race woman comes to your clinic complaining of back pain and bowing of her legs that she has had since childhood. She has been taking over the counter vitamin D supplements to no avail.

Care of acutely ill patients

A. IM Epinephrine
B. Benzylpenicillin
C. Oxygen
D. Aspirin
E. Nebulized Salbutamol
F. Glucagon
G. IV fluids
H. IV Lorazepam
I. Insulin sliding scale
J. Admit to Hospital
K. Refer for urgent mental health assessment
L. PO Lorazepam
M. Defibrillation
N. Refer for urgent eye clinic appointment

For each case below, select the **SINGLE MOST** appropriate answer from the options above. Each option can be used once, more than once or not at all.

66. You are asked to see a 13 year old girl at her home. She has been sent home from school with severe abdominal pain. She now has a headache that is made worse by light and has a diffuse rash that blanches with pressure.

67. You are completing your round of the local nursing home when a nurse leads you to Roy's room. This morning he has become increasingly confused and is now having visual hallucinations and behaving violently toward the staff. The nursing-staff are unable to look after him in his present state.

68. A 50 year old man with recently diagnosed heart failure presents with shortness of breath, wheeze and a swollen face. He collapses in your surgery.

69. An 80 year old patient on your ward has become acutely confused and is refusing to eat or drink. On examination she is hypotensive with tachycardia and smells strongly of urine.

70. A 20 year old woman has collapsed after a sprinting session at her local athletics club. On examination she is not breathing and you can't detect a pulse, her GCS is 3/15. Her brother died suddenly 3 years ago.

Digestive problems – Pancreatic disease

A. Alcohol
B. Unknown
C. Post-ERCP
D. Mycoplasma infection
E. Gallstones
F. Drugs
G. Viral infection
H. Pancreatic tumour
I. Hyperlipidaemia
J. Pregnancy
K. Scorpion sting

For each case below, select the **SINGLE MOST** appropriate answer from the options above. Each option can be used once, more than once or not at all.

71. A 50 year old patient with a history of past alcohol abuse, diabetes and a 20 pack year history presents with constant gnawing pain in his abdomen radiating to his back.

72. A 30 year old woman presents with sudden onset of very severe abdominal pain and vomiting. She strongly denies excessive drinking and her last menstrual period was 2 weeks ago.

73. A 50 year old biker presents with an acute abdomen. He smells strongly of alcohol and admits to past intravenous drug use.

74. A 48 year old West Indian man presents with acute pancreatitis. On his chest X-ray you note bilateral hilar lymphadenopathy. He tells you that this was noted years ago and he is now receiving treatment for a chronic disease.

75. A 54 year old woman is brought in with severe abdominal pain. Over the last 3 months she has begun to lose weight. She says she has no interest in eating or socialising since the death of her husband. You notice that she has been admitted five times this year with falls.

Respiratory problems – Chest infections

A. Co-Amoxiclav PO
B. Oxygen PRN
C. Doxycycline PO
D. Urgent admission to hospital
E. Erythromycin PO
F. Co-Amoxiclav and Clarithromycin IV
G. Consider hospital referral
H. Nebulized Salbutamol
I. Tazobactam-Piperacillin IV
J. Ciprofloxacin PO
K. Prednisolone PO

For each case below, select the **SINGLE MOST** appropriate answer from the options above. Each option can be used once, more than once or not at all.

76. An 80 year old patient presents with a three day history of a cough productive of green sputum. There are a few crackles in her right lung base but her blood pressure and respiratory rate are normal.

77. A 50 year old man with asthma presents with a productive cough, green sputum and pleuritic chest pain. He is mildly confused, has a respiratory rate of 30 and a blood pressure of 90/67mmHg and he is allergic to Penicillin.

78. A 73 year old woman presents with a 4 day history of cough and green sputum. She has a blood pressure of 100/62, a respiratory rate of 20 and is mildly confused. She has crackles in her left lung base.

79. A 63 year old with COPD complains of increased thick yellow sputum and shortness of breath. He is allergic to Penicillin.

80. A 34 year old woman has recently returned from hospital after a complicated labour. Her child has spent 3 days on the neonatal unit but is now home. She complains of chest pain, cough and green sputum. You see her in the A+E department.

Care of children and young people

A. Desmopressin
B. Developmental delay
C. Trimethoprim
D. School nurse
E. Enuresis alarm
F. Encoparesis
G. Constipation
H. Nocturnal enuresis
I. No action
J. Peadiatrician referral
K. Paroxetine

For each case below, select the **SINGLE MOST** appropriate answer from the options above. Each option can be used once, more than once or not at all.

81. A mother of a 5 year old boy presents with you complaining that he is still wetting the bed.

82. A 7 year old girl has been brought to your clinic because she has begun to smell of faeces and has constantly soiled knickers. Her mother wants to know what has caused this.

83. A 7 year old boy is still wetting the bed. His mother has tried many things and now wants to be referred for further help.

84. An 11 year old boy has begun to wet the bed again. This has started to make him feel sad especially as he can no longer sleep over at his friend's house.

85. A previously continent 5 year old girl has presented with her third urinary tract infection.

Cardiovascular problems – Management of chest pain

A. Myocardial infarction
B. Pneumothorax
C. Costochondritis
D. Myocarditis
E. Pericarditis
F. Pulmonary embolism
G. Gastro-oesophageal reflux disease
H. Anxiety
I. Shingles
J. Dissecting aortic aneurysm
K. Pneumonia

For each case described, select the **SINGLE MOST** appropriate diagnosis from the options above. Each option may be used once, more than once or not at all.

86. A 28 year old man has a 3 day history of fever and a sharp, central, constant stabbing chest pain. The pain is worse on deep inspiration and relieved by bending forwards. On examination, his temperature is 38.8°C and cardio-respiratory examination is normal.

87. A 30 year old woman presents with a sudden onset of left, sharp chest pain which is worse on deep inspiration. She also feels short of breath on moderate exertion. She takes the oral combined contraceptive pill and is a non-smoker.

88. A 70 year old man presents with a two hour history of left sided chest pain radiating to his left shoulder. He also feels a bit clammy and nauseous. He had a stroke two years ago and is still smoking 40 cigarettes per day.

89. A tall, 19 year old male presents with sudden onset of shortness of breath and right sided chest pain which is worse on deep inspiration. He is known to have asthma but says this is unlike his usual asthma attacks, as he is not 'wheezy' at all.

90. An 18 year old female has a 7 day history of chest tightness, which is worst at night. There is no associated shortness of breath, wheeze or radiation. She has known irritable bowel syndrome and has her A-level exams next week. Cardio-respiratory examination, ECG and chest X-ray are all normal.

Neurological problems – Stroke anatomy

A. Left-sided lacunar infarct
B. Right-sided brainstem infarct
C. Left internal carotid artery infarct
D. Right anterior cerebral artery infarct
E. Right middle cerebral artery infarct
F. Left anterior inferior cerebellar artery infarct
G. Right external carotid artery infarct
I. Left posterior cerebral artery infarct
J. Right posterior inferior cerebellar artery infarct
K. Left vertebral artery infarct

For each set of stroke symptoms described in each case, select the **SINGLE MOST** appropriate vascular territory of the brain affected from the list above. Each option may be used once, more than once or not at all.

91. A right-handed, 80 year old woman presents with weakness of the left side of her face, tongue and left arm (with relative sparing of her left leg). She also has sensory neglect of her left arm and leg and problems with dressing herself.

92. A 75 year old man presents with in-coordination and unsteadiness in his right leg and right arm. He also complains of problems swallowing and 'the room spinning around'. On examination, he also has nystagmus.

93. A 66 year old woman complains of a progressively worsening weakness and sensory disturbance of her right arm and right leg. She also has a left-sided frontal headache. On examination, she has a bruit audible on auscultation on the left side of her neck.

94. A 71 year old man presents with weakness and sensory loss which is much worse in his left leg compared to his left arm. He has also lost his sense of smell and his wife has noticed he has become surprisingly sexually disinhibited.

95. A 91 year old woman presents with loss of the right half of her vision in both eyes.

Skin problems – Rashes

A. Pityriasis rosea
B. Seborrhoeic keratosis
C. Erythema nodosum
D. Vitiligo
E. Keratosis pilaris
F. Erythema multiforme
G. Molluscum contagiosum
H. Pityriasis versicolor
I. Tinea cruris
J. Scabies
K. Chickenpox

For each rash described, select the **SINGLE MOST** appropriate diagnosis from the options above. Each option may be used once, more than once or not at all.

96. An 8 year old boy presents with pearly, umbilicated papules on his chest and arms. He is asymptomatic. Mum remembers his sister has a couple of similar lesions on her trunk too.

97. A 12 year old girl presents with a 'goose-pimple' rash on her arms and legs, with small, red papules around the hair follicles. The rash is easier to feel than to see and she also has atopic eczema. She is asymptomatic.

98. A 16 year old boy presents with pink, oval-shaped lesions (1-3cm diameter) with a scaly edge on his back, chest and abdomen. He remembers the rash began as just a single oval lesion on his abdomen and then became widespread 10–15 days later. The lesions run parallel with his skin creases. He is asymptomatic.

99. A 20 year old Caucasian woman noticed some small, pale patches on her chest and back a few weeks ago, which suddenly become much more noticeable after going on a sunny holiday to Greece. The rash is slightly itchy at times.

100. A 25 year old rugby player has erupted in a very itchy rash on her groins. She has small, circular patches with a red, scaly edge and a paler centre. Some of the lesions have joined together. She admits to occasionally sharing towels.

Answer section: Extended Match Questions

1. G

   Niacin, also called nicotinic acid, is a water soluble vitamin derived from the amino acid tryptophan. It is found in meat, liver, fish, whole-grain products and beans. Niacin deficiency causes these symptoms of dermatitis, dementia, diarrhoea and also death. This is called pellagra. Treatment for this is with nicotinic acid.

2. B

   Vitamin C is a water soluble compound which helps promotes many metabolic reactions including the laying down of collagen during connective tissue formation and it also promotes wound healing. It is found in citrus fruits, green vegetables, milk and liver. Vitamin C deficiency causes scurvy (rare in developed countries).In scurvy the person has anaemia, bleeding gums and teeth, bruising and poor wound healing. Treatment is with vitamin C.

3. H

   Vitamin B6 (pyridoxine) is a water soluble vitamin found in salmon, tomatoes, whole-grain products and yoghurt. It is an essential coenzyme for many reactions. It is associated with malabsorption and drug antagonists of vitamin B6. Features of Vitamin B6 deficiency include mental confusion, inflammation of the mouth, tongue and eyes and also peripheral neuropathy. Treatment is with Vitamin B6.

4. J

   Folate is present in most foods, notably green vegetables, liver and nuts. Deficiency is associated with macrocytic anaemia, glossitis, malabsorption and subacute combined degeneration of the cord. Folic acid is given at the time of conception to help prevent neural tube defects.

5. A

Vitamin A is a fat soluble vitamin found in liver, butter, cheese and fruits and vegetables. Deficiency of this causes atrophy and keratinisation of the epithelium. Symptoms include dry skin and hair, drying of the cornea, nervous disorders and also night blindness. Treatment includes Vitamin A supplements.

6. F

Peppermint oil is used for Irritable Bowel Syndrome

7. A

8. D

Saw palmetto treats Benign Prostatic Hypertrophy
St. John's Wort is used for depression

9. C

Feverfew is for migraines

10. B

Echinacea is for the common cold

11. A

Fibroadenomas are a common and benign condition. They are common in women <35 years old. They present with a painless, hard, mobile lump which often slips as you try to examine it hence their name as a breast mouse. Diagnosis is by clinical assessment, ultrasound and fine needle aspiration. In women under 40 excision is not required unless the lump is >4cm in diameter. In women over 40 all lumps should be excised.

12. C

This is a classic description of a breast cancer especially in view of her family history. Breast cancer is the most common malignancy in women with 1 in 11 suffering from it in their lifetime. Risk factors include previous breast cancer, female sex, family history, early menarche or late menopause, nulliparity or first child when >30, Caucasian, age, obesity, alcohol, previous ovarian and endometrial cancer. It can be asymptomatic but presents with a palpable breast lump (40–50% in upper outer quadrant), skin tethering, Paget's disease of the breast, Peau d'orange, nipple inversion or discharge. There can also be lymphadenopathy and other signs of metastases such as bone pain and jaundice. Investigations include ultrasound, mammography and fine needle aspiration and others such as CT scan to exclude spread. Treatment includes surgery, radiotherapy and chemotherapy.

13. G

Fat necrosis can follow a trivial injury and cause pain. On examination, there may be a hard, irregular lump which can become tethered to the skin. It can be hard to distinguish this from malignancy so excision biopsy may be needed to exclude it with certainty.

14. F

Breast abscess is common in lactating women following mastitis. It presents with a hot, tender, swollen breast and the patient may be unwell. Antibiotics may help but drainage may also be needed.

15. E

Duct ectasia is dilatation of the large and intermediate breast ducts. It is common in women around the age of menopause and above. It presents with a hard or doughy tender lump beneath or close to the areola and with nipple discharge which can be cheesy or green or blood stained. There can also be some slit-like nipple retraction. If there is infection then antibiotics can be used, if there is a collection then drainage, and sometimes surgery may be needed.

16. B

Miscarriage is the spontaneous discharge of the gestation sac before the foetus is viable up to 24 weeks. Eighty percent happen in the first 12 weeks. Risk factors are smoking, maternal age and alcohol. Threatened miscarriage is when there is vaginal bleeding but the cervical os is closed and there is no loss of products of conception. The uterus is normal size for dates. There may be some abdominal discomfort and foetal heart and movements are fine.

17. A

Inevitable miscarriage is when there is bleeding, abdominal pain, and the cervical os is open.

18. H

This is a stillbirth as it is after 24 weeks gestation.

19. D

Missed miscarriage is when there are few symptoms, the cervical os is closed and the uterus is smaller than expected. Referral should be done for an early pregnancy scan and management can be either conservative or surgical with evacuation of retained products of conception.

20. G

Ectopic pregnancy occurs when the products of conception implant outside the uterus, most often in the fallopian tube. This diagnosis should be considered in any woman of reproductive age who complains of abdominal pain. Risk factors include previous ectopic, previous tubal surgery, Pelvic Inflammatory Disease, Intrauterine Device insitu. The woman will have amenorrhoea (seven weeks is peak incidence), abdominal pain in most cases which may radiate to the shoulder tip and also vaginal bleeding. Immediate referral to hospital for further management is needed. Options include expectant, medical with methotrexate and surgical with laparoscopy or laparotomy.

21. D

A Med 6 is used when it is felt putting a diagnosis on a Med 3 or 4 would be harmful to the patient. It is then sent to the Department of Works and Pensions who will send a form to obtain more accurate information.

22. B

A Med 4 is usually requested by the Department of Work and Pensions after a patient has had 28 weeks of incapacity to confirm the nature of the condition and to undergo a Personal Capability Assessment.

23. F

A SC2 is for people who can claim statutory sick pay. SC1 is a self certificate for those not eligible for statutory sick pay.

24. A

For a Med 3, the doctor must examine the patient on the day or day before the note is issued. It can be a closed certificate or open (one month initially). Before the patient returns to work you should reassess and give a further certificate with date of return.

25. H

A DS 1500 form is for patients that are terminally ill. It should be given to the patient or their representative and not to the Department of Work and Pensions directly. It asks for factual information and does not require a prognosis.

26. F

This is when the nucleus pulposus squeezes through the annulus fibrosis and bulges in a posterior or posterolateral direction. This causes pressure on the nerve root below the herniation, most commonly S1, L5 and then L4. It presents with sudden onset back pain with very limited movement. There is pain in the leg and buttock and there may be paraesthesia or numbness in the leg or foot.

27. E

A multiple myeloma is a malignant neoplasm of plasma cells that arises in the bone marrow. Presentation is with anaemia, renal failure, infection, hypercalcaemia, bone pain, pathologic fractures, or Bence Jones proteinuria and high ESR. Incidence increases with age. The main sites for myeloma involvement are the proximal long bones, the pelvis, the thoracic cage, the vertebral column and the skull. Treatment includes supportive measures and chemotherapy.

28. D
Ankylosing spondylitis is a seronegative arthropathy. It is more common in male Caucasians compared to females in a ratio of 3:1. 95% of cases are HLA B27 positive. It typically presents with morning back pain/stiffness in young men. Associated symptoms include decreased chest expansion, hip and knee arthritis, iritis, plantar fasciitis, Crohn's disease, Ulcerative Colitis, osteoporosis, psoriaform rashes and aortic regurgitation. The ESR is elevated and there may be vertebral squaring and fusion of the spine (bamboo spine). Management is with exercise, NSAIDs and referral to rheumatology.

29. C
Osteoarthritis is a metabolically active disease involving the whole joint in which you get loss of articular cartilage and overgrowth of the underlying bone. It is more common in women and also in Afro-Carribean and Asian people. Patients get joint pain and stiffness, crepitus, and decreased function. It most commonly affects the hips, knees and base of the thumb. X-rays show a loss of joint space, cysts, subchondral sclerosis and osteophytes. Management is with pain control and exercise.

30. H
Sinister features such as weight loss and back pain suggest a malignancy.

31. D
This man has an enlarged prostate on examination and his PSA result is higher than what the normal range is for his age. This indicates that prostate cancer is the most likely option from the list.

32. E
Benign Prostatic Hypertrophy is common in elderly men and presents with lower urinary tract symptoms. The PSA in this case is not very high and so this makes malignancy less likely.

33. A
Testicular torsion is a surgical emergency. It is most common in adolescents. It typically presents with a swollen, painful scrotum and abdominal pain, sometimes vomiting. There may be a history of mild trauma. Pain is not relieved by lifting the twisted testis (negative Prehn's sign). In epididymitis elevation relieves pain. Treatment is with urgent surgery.

34. C

Testicular cancer is the most common malignancy in men aged between 20–34. Risk factors include having undescended testes and a past history of testicular cancer. Presentation is with a painless lump (may be pain also), and there may be other symptoms such as back pain if there are metastases. Urgent urological opinion is needed and treatment depends on tumour type and extent of spread.

35. F

UTI in men are less common than in women. The positive urine dipstick for nitrites and leucocytes as well as the symptom of dysuria make this the most likely diagnosis. Further investigations involving blood tests and also imaging should be done to establish the cause.

36. B

Pain worse on exertion is common in Osteoarthritis as is the x-ray finding of reduced joint space.

37. D

The World Health Organisation has defined osteoporosis as a bone mineral density T score on DEXA scan more than 2.5 standard deviations below the mean.

38. H

Osteopaenia is defined as having a bone density 1 to 2.5 standard deviations below the mean (T score –1 to –2.5).

39. A

Septic arthritis is inflammation within a joint space most commonly as a result of haematogenous spread. It occurs most commonly in children, the elderly or the immunosuppressed. It usually affects one joint (mostly hip or knee) and presents with a painful, swollen, red, hot joint. Movement of the joint is limited and there may be a temperature and tachycardia. Investigations include a full blood count and inflammatory markers, blood cultures and joint aspiration of fluid. Patient should be admitted urgently to hospital and commenced on IV antibiotics.

40. G

Psoriatic arthritis is a seronegative arthropathy. It causes pain, swelling and stiffness of the joints. The main types include an oligoarthritis, symmetrical polyarthritis indistinguishable from rheumatoid arthritis, arthritis mutilans, psoriatic spondylitis and distal interphalangeal arthritis with nail dystrophy.

41. C

Berne (1964); *'Games People Play.'* Doctors and their patients may assume different roles such as parent and child. The key is to recognise what roles the patient and yourself are playing.

42. G

Helman (1981, 2007) Folk Model – What has happened? Why has it happened? Why has it happened to me? Why now? What would happen if nothing was done about it? What are the likely effects on the other people around me? What should I do and where can I seek help?

43. I

Pendleton *et al* – Read *'The New Consultation'*

44. H

Heron (1975, 1989) *'Six category intervention analysis.'* A doctor can use prescriptive, informative, cathartic, catalytic, supportive and confrontational interventions with patients.

45. J

Neighbour (1987, 2004) – Read *'The inner consultation'*

46. A

The Incident Decision Tree is a useful tool on the NPSA website.

47. E

This is an honest mistake and should be reported to the MHRA.

48. I

Unless multi-source feedback forms are completed honestly they are no use to the doctor or their patients.

49. C

Improving staff training will most directly prevent this event from recurring. Answer D 'Being open and fair' will help but not as much as answer C.

50. H

Performing an audit of patients on Spironolactone to ascertain how many have had their U & E's checked within the required time period will directly help to prevent this from happening again. A Significant Events Analysis will help but an audit can show how many patients are not being monitored adequately instead of focusing on one incident.

51. H

Fathers are permitted 2 weeks paid paternity leave following the birth of their child or on adoption. Furthermore adoptive parents are permitted 52 weeks parental leave, 39 of which are paid.

52. G

This act means that GP principals have a legal responsibility to actively pursue reasonable measures to prevent discrimination of disabled patients through making sure they can access the practice.

53. B

Race Relations Act 1976 prevents discrimination in any public body on grounds of race or nationality.

54. D

The Sexual Discrimination Act prevents women being unfairly disadvantaged at interviews. Sometimes acts of discrimination can be mistaken for valid concerns about the cost of employing certain employees.

55. A

The Race Relations Amendment Act 2000 means that public institutions must not only prevent racial discrimination but positively promote equality and the prevention of racial discrimination. Thus there can be questions regarding race when applying for jobs in order to prove equality of access to jobs offered however there must be a policy to promote racial equality and prevent discrimination.

56. A

57. D

58. B

59. E

60. I

Try to memorise the dates of major milestones in childhood development in the four categories: Gross motor skills, Fine motor and adaptive skills, language and personal/social skills

61. D

Robertsonian Translocation occurs when the there is the transfer of genetic information between the long and short arms of chromosomes 14 and 21. These 'translocations' can result with male gametes containing either normal quantities of chromosomes, balanced translocations, unbalanced translocations or missing chromosomes.

62. K

This is Angelman syndrome which is due to an interstitial deletion of a region of chromosome 15 inherited from the maternal line and is an example of imprinting. However, when this mutation is inherited from the paternal line the disease caused is Prader-Willi syndrome which consists of obesity, short stature, hypogonadism and learning difficulties.

63. E

Anticipation occurs in autosomal dominant disorders when there is expansion of an unstable triplet repeat sequences. Replication of the CAG neucleotide triplet has been demonstrated to be associated with an increased risk of juvenile Huntington's disease.

64. H

Babies with Patau's syndrome rarely survive and when they do their prognosis is very poor.

65. I

Vitamin D resistant rickets is one of the few X linked dominant disease.

66. B

Bacterial meningitis can present with abdominal pain and meningococcal septicaemia can present with a blanching rash before the distinctive purpuric rash. Clinical acumen is therefore vital and if meningitis, or meningoccal septicaemia are diagnoses' in your differential then these patients should be given IM Benzylpenicillin and admitted to hospital.

67. J

This patient has an acute confusional state. The most common cause of this is infection. This is an indication to admit a patient. One to one nursing in a side room with adequate lighting is indicated for these patients.

68. A

This patient has angioedema due to starting Ramipril for his heart failure and is having an anaphylactic attack. Check his ABC's, give IM adrenaline/epinephrine and call 999.

69. G

This patient is dehydrated due to a UTI. Do not treat her acute confusional state without addressing the cause of this.

70. J

This patient probably has hypertrophic obstructive cardiomyopathy. Even if she does not, she is in cardiac arrest and if her heart arrhythmia is either ventricular tachycardia or fibrillation then she should receive defibrillation as soon as possible. In some countries an echocardiogram is performed prior to any potential athlete being allowed to train.

71. H

Risk factors for pancreatic carcinoma include excessive alcohol consumption, diabetes and smoking. The prognosis is very poor and when occurring in the head of the pancreas is associated with painless jaundice.

72. E

Alcohol and gallstones account for 80% of cases of pancreatitis.

73. G

HIV affects many different people and the key risk factor to consider is unsafe practices.

74. F

Sarcoidosis is treated with steroids and often steroid sparing drugs such as Azathioprine which can cause pancreatitis.

75. A

As for question 72, Alcohol is a common cause and pancreatitis should be a differential in any heavy drinker with abdominal pain.

76. A

The CURB65 score: (C = CONFUSION, U = Raised urea, R = Raised respiratory rate (≥30), B = Blood pressure ≤90 systolic/≥60 systolic). A CURB65 of 0 means the patient can probably be treated at home.

77. D

CURB65 = 3 needs urgent referral to hospital

78. G

CURB65 = 2 consider hospital admission

79. C

Infective COPD exacerbation

80. F

She may have hospital acquired pneumonia

81. I

Children aged ≤6 who wet the bed will usually grow out of it. Reassure the parent and offer constructive advice.

82. F

This is encoparesis which can be caused by constipation, developmental delay and behavioural problems. These patients should be referred to the paediatric developmental clinic.

83. D

The school nurse is usually very experienced in helping children with these problems.

84. A

This will help him when over at a friend's house and can be used with other techniques to promote nocturnal continence.

85. J

She needs to have an urgent urinary USS to exclude vesicouretal reflux (VUR). This condition results in the retrograde flow of urine from the bladder to the kidneys and causes recurrent urinary tract infections, pyelonephritis and later hypotension and progressive renal failure.

86. E
Pericarditis – mostly viral and characterised by sharp pain (may be pleuritic) - worse on lying down and relieved by bending forwards. Also due to TB, post-MI (Dressler's syndrome), renal failure (uraemia), trauma, connective tissue disorders (e.g. SLE), hypothyroidism, pneumonia/septicaemia

87. F
Pulmonary embolism – sudden onset dyspnoea and pleuritic chest pain. Is there calf pain/swelling? Presence of any risk factors: Combined pill use/recent immobility or surgery/malignancy?

88. A
Myocardial infarction – typical cardiac sounding chest pain, but elderly and diabetics can get 'silent MIs' without chest pain. Is there any relief with GTN? Do they have any cardiovascular risk factors?

89. B
Pneumothorax – sudden onset dyspnoea and pleuritic chest pain. This is more common in tall, slim males and also in asthmatics and Marfan's.

90. H
Anxiety – anxiety may present as vague chest pains, but anxiety would be a diagnosis of exclusion (once serious causes of chest pain have been ruled out)

91. E
Middle cerebral artery infarct – presents with contralateral hemiplegia (face, tongue, arm>leg) and neglect of contralateral limb if non-dominant hemisphere affected and global dysphasia if non-dominant hemisphere affected.

92. I
Posterior inferior cerebellar artery infarct – ipsilateral limb ataxia, vertigo, vomiting, nystagmus.

93. C
Internal carotid artery infarct – carotid bruit, unilateral frontal headache, progressing contralateral hemiplegia and hemisensory disturbance, contralateral homonymous hemianopia, deteriorating consciousness.

94. D

Anterior cerebral artery infarct – can present with contralateral hemiplegia and hemisensory loss (leg>arm) and behavioural changes.

95. H

Posterior cerebral artery infarct – occlusion of cortical vessels can produce a homonymous hemianopia.

96. G

Molluscum contagiosum – rash caused by a DNA pox virus which is characterised by firm, round umbilicated papules containing caseous material and is common in children.

97. E

Keratosis pilaris – characterised by small follicular plugs and red papules which usually occur on the arms thighs and face.

98. A

Pityriasis rosea – self-limiting rash presumed to be due to human herpes virus 7 (HHV7), usually presenting as a single, oval, 2–3 cm diameter, scaly plaque on the trunk ('herald patch'). A few days later, similar (but smaller) lesions erupt on the limbs and trunk in a 'Christmas tree' distribution along the line creases. More common in children and young adolescents.

99. H

Pityriasis versicolor – yeast infection (most commonly due to Malassezzia furfur), which presents as scaly, depigmented lesions < 1 cm diameter, which become more noticeable when the rest of the skin becomes tanned.

100. I

Tinea cruris – or 'jock itch' is ringworm or fungal infection of the groins (due to Microphyton, Trichophyton and Epidermophyton species), characterised by pink papules with a scaly edge and central clearing.

Picture Question Paper

Cardiovascular problems – Hypertension questions 1–5

For each of the numbered gaps in Figure 1, please select **ONE** of the options from the list below. Each option may be used once, more than once or not at all.

Figure 1 is adapted from the NICE quick reference guidelines on the management of hypertension:

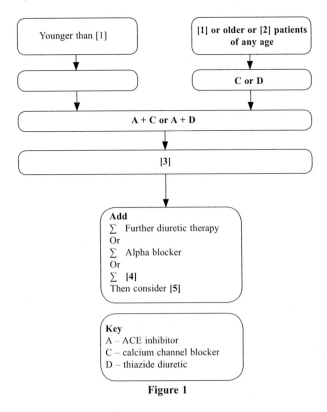

Figure 1

A. 55 years old
B. 65 years old
C. Chinese
D. Caucasian
E. Black
F. Seeking specialist advice
G. Angiotensin-II receptor antagonist + calcium channel blocker + thiazide diuretic
H. ACE inhibitor + calcium channel blocker + thiazide diuretic
I. Beta Blocker
J. Minoxidil

1. Blank 1   A
2. Blank 2   E
3. Blank 3   H
4. Blank 4   I
5. Blank 5   F

Skin problems – Rash

6. A 12 year old girl presents with a rapidly worsening, painful rash on her face (see Figure 2) which involves crops of blisters which look like cold sores. She also has circular, punched-out erosions and worsening red, dry, flaky, weepy skin on her face. She has had eczema previously as a child.

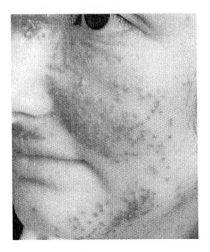

Figure 2

What is the **SINGLE MOST** likely diagnosis? Select **ONE** option only.

   A. Ophthalmic shingles
   B. Herpes zoster
   C. Eczema herpeticum
   D. Measles
   E. Molluscum contagiosum

Skin problems – Lesion

7. A 28 year old woman says she has had this mole on her back for many years (see Figure 3), but feels its shape has changed over the last few weeks. She is fair-skinned, enjoys going on sunny holidays and admits to using sun-beds in the past.

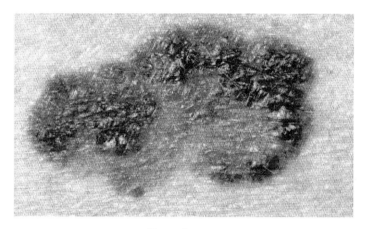

Figure 3

What is the **SINGLE MOST** likely diagnosis? Select **ONE** option only.

A. Benign compound naevus
B. Seborrhoeic keratosis
C. Pigmented nodular basal cell carcinoma
D. Malignant melanoma
E. Pyogenic granuloma

Research & academic activity – Data representation

8. What is the name for the type of data representation shown in Figure 4? Select **ONE** option only.

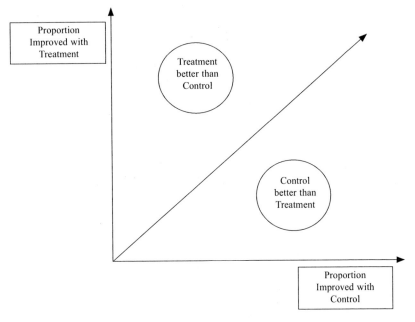

Figure 4

A. Box and whisker plot
B. Bar chart
C. Pie chart
D. Forest plot
E. L'Abbé plot

visual representation comparing treatment to placebo

Skin problems – Rash

9. This 28 year old man with mild acne vulgaris on his back (see Figure 5), presents to you with a few pink papules, blackheads and whiteheads on his upper back, with no scarring. He has already tried over the counter treatments including benzoyl peroxide which did not have any effect.

Figure 5

Which is the **SINGLE MOST INAPPROPRIATE** next step of treatment? Select **ONE** option only.

A. Higher concentration benzoyl peroxide
B. Topical retinoid
C. Oral retinoid
D. Topical antibiotic + benzoyl peroxide
E. Azelaic acid

Women's health – Management of menorrhagia

10. For Figure 6 below, regarding the management of fibroids, which is adapted from the NICE quick reference guidelines on heavy menstrual bleeding, what is the missing box X? Select **ONE** option only.

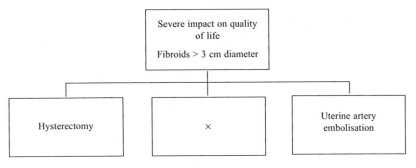

Figure 6

    A. Dilatation and curettage
    B. Hysteroscopy
    C. Endometrial ablation
    D. Myomectomy
    E. None of the above

Genetics in primary care questions 11–15

Please look at Figure 7 below. For each question below, select the **SINGLE MOST** appropriate option from the list below. Each option can be used once, more than once or not at all.

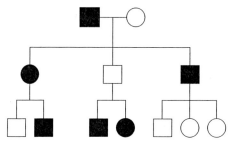

Figure 7

A. X-linked recessive
B. Autosomal dominant
C. Adult onset polycystic kidney disease
D. Robertsonian translocation
E. Anticipation
F. Incomplete penetrance
G. Autosomal recessive
H. Haemophilia
I. X-linked dominant
J. Vitamin D resistant rickets
K. Imprinting

11. What is the mode of inheritance of disease in the diagram above?
12. What form of altered expression is demonstrated in the diagram?
13. What would be the term given to this type of genetic disorder if it got worse with each generation of sufferers?
14. What would be the term given to this type of genetic disorder if the symptoms and signs were dependent on whether the gene was maternally or paternally inherited?
15. What could this disorder be?

ENT & facial problems – Nose problem

16. What is the condition shown in Figure 8? Select **ONE** option only.

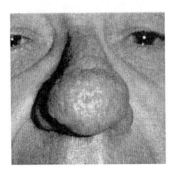

Figure 8

A. Marfan's syndrome
B. Basal cell carcinoma
C. Squamous cell carcinoma
D. Acromegaly
E. Rhinophyma

The general practice xonsultation questions 17–21

For each numbered blank space in Figure 9 below, select the correct answer from the options below. Each option can be used once, more than once or not at all.

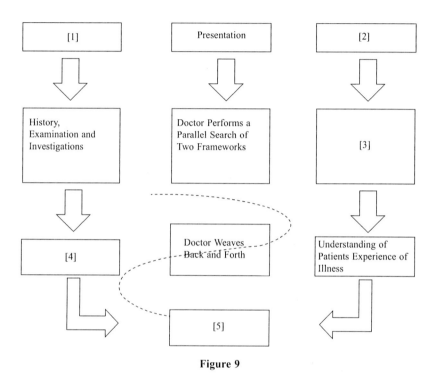

Figure 9

A. Active listening
B. Illness framework
C. Exploring Health beliefs
D. Ideas, concerns and expectations
E. Non-verbal cues
F. Integrated Understanding
G. Referral
H. Differential Diagnosis
I. Disease Framework
J. Management plan
K. Feedback

17. Blank 1
18. Blank 2
19. Blank 3
20. Blank 4
21. Blank 5

Research & academic activity – Data distribution

22. Which of the following statements is **TRUE** about Graph 1 below?
     Select **ONE** option only.

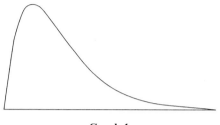

Graph 1

A. Mean = median = mode
B. Mean < median < mode
C. Mean > median > mode
D. Mean < mode < median
E. Median < mode < mean

Skin problems – Rash

23. A 65 year old woman has developed a red rash on her cheeks and nose over the last few months (see Figure 10). She drinks 30 units per week and feels that alcohol does make the rash worse. On examination, she has erythema in the areas described earlier, with some papules and pustules on her nose and telangiectasia on her cheeks.

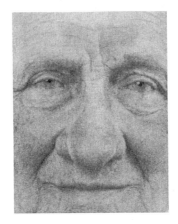

Figure 10

Which is the **SINGLE MOST** likely diagnosis? Select **ONE** option only.

A. Systemic lupus erythematosus
B. Side-effect of increased alcohol intake
C. Acnea rosacea
D. Acne vulgaris
E. Seborrhoeic dermatitis

Respiratory problems – SIGN/BTS guidance for adults questions 24–28

For each numbered blank space in the diagram below select the correct answer from the options below. Each option can be used once, more than once or not at all.

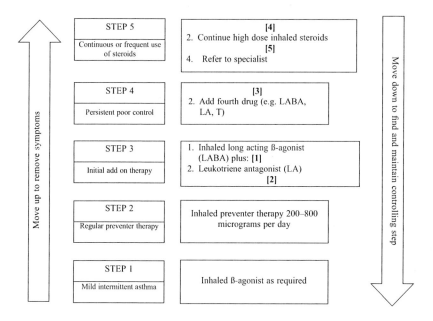

Figure 11

A. Montelukast 10 mg nocte
B. Salbutamol 100 micrograms
C. Nebulised Ipratropium bromide
D. Lowest effective dose prednisolone
E   Beclomethasone 400 micrograms
F. Steroid sparing medication
G. Beclomethasone 800 micrograms
H. High-dose prednisolone
I. Uniphyllin
J. Magnesium sulphate
K. Beclomethasone 2000 micrograms

24. Blank 1
25. Blank 2
26. Blank 3
27. Blank 4
28. Blank 5

Digestive problems – Liver function tests

29. A 30 year old woman has a raised Body Mass Index (BMI) of 39. She does not drink any alcohol, has not been abroad recently and is not on any regular medications. The results of some routine liver function tests are shown in Table 1 below:

Full blood count		Normal
Bilirubin	10 μmol/L	(0 – 17 μmol/L)
Alkaline Phosphatase (ALP)	167 u/L	(100 – 300 u/L)
Aspartate Transaminase (AST)	48 iu/L	(5 – 42 iu/L)
Alanine Transaminase (ALT)	64 iu/L	(5 – 42 iu/L)
Gamma gluteryl transaminase (GGT)	38 iu/L	(5 – 30 iu/L)

Table 1

What is the **SINGLE MOST** likely diagnosis? Select **ONE** option only.

A. Alcoholic liver disease
B. Fatty liver infiltration
C. Gall stones
D. Viral hepatitis
E. Hepatic malignancy

Digestive problems – Rectal bleeding

30. A 70 year old woman, with known haemorrhoids, presents with minor
     fresh rectal bleeding (noticed on wiping) for 3 days. Apart from
     a small external haemorrhoid, rectal and abdominal examinations
     are normal. The results of some routine blood tests are shows in
     Table 2 below:

Haemoglobin	9.1 g/dL	(12.0 – 15.0 g/dL)
White cell count	10.3 x10^9/L	(4.0 – 11.0 x 10^9/L)
Platelets	338 x 10^9/L	(150 – 400 x 10^9/L)
Mean Corpuscular Volume	70 fL	(80 – 100 fL)
Ferritin	10 μg/L	(14 – 200 μg/L)

Table 2

Select the SINGLE MOST appropriate next step of management
from the options below. Select ONE option only.

A. Give 3 months of oral iron therapy
B. Treat with topical therapy for haemorrhoids
C. Observe + monitor for 'red flag' symptoms such as weight
    loss, change in bowel habit, etc.
D. Refer urgently to colorectal clinic on a 14-day referral for
    suspected cancer
E. Refer routinely to colorectal clinic for treatment of haemorrhoids
    (e.g. for banding)

Sexual health – Vaginal discharge

Using Table 3 below, which is about different types of vaginal discharge, fill in the missing blanks using the options listed below. Select **ONE** option only.

	Bacterial vaginosis	Candida	Trichomonas vaginalis
Symptoms	[1] Offensive fishy odour No itch	Thick white discharge [2] Vulval itch or soreness Superficial dyspareunia External dysuria	[3] Offensive Vulval itch Dysuria Abdominal pain
Signs	Discharge coating vagina and vestibule No vulval inflammation	Normal findings or Vulval erythema, oedema, fissuring, satellite lesions	Vulvitis and vaginitis So called [4]
pH	[5]	<4.5	≥4.5

Table 3

    A. Thin discharge
    B. ≥4.5
    C. Non-offensive discharge
    D. Scanty to profuse or frothy yellow discharge
    E. <4.5
    F. Strawberry cervix
    G. Vaginal bleeding
    H. 4.5

31. Blank 1
32. Blank 2
33. Blank 3
34. Blank 4
35. Blank 5

Skin problems – Rash

36. A 23 year old male has had a sore throat for the last 2 days and has now developed an itchy rash over his body. On examination, he has several small, salmon-pink, dew drop papules over his trunk and also on his limbs (see Figure 12 below).

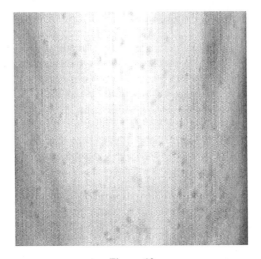

Figure 12

Select the **SINGLE MOST** likely diagnosis from the list below. Select **ONE** option only.

A. Pityriasis versicolor
B. Pityriasis rosea
C. Chronic stable plaque psoriasis
D. Meningococcal septicaemia
E. Guttate psoriasis

Neurological problems – Facial weakness

37. An 18 year old student visits the surgery as she woke up this morning and found that the left side of her face was 'paralysed' (see Figure 13 below). She has also lost her sense of smell, finds loud sounds uncomfortable and has a pain around her left ear. On examination, she has a left facial droop and cannot close her left eye or wrinkle the left side of her forehead. Examination of the peripheral nervous system is normal and so is ear, nose and throat examination.

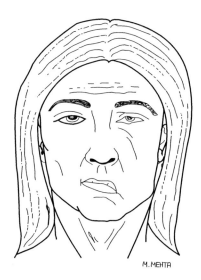

M.MEHTA

Figure 13

Select the **SINGLE MOST** likely diagnosis. Select **ONE** option only,

A. Parotid tumour
B. Stroke
C. Ramsay-Hunt syndrome
D. Multiple sclerosis
E. Bell's palsy

Respiratory problems - SIGN/BTS guidelines for asthma in children aged 5–12 years questions 38–42

For each numbered blank space in the diagram below select the correct answer from the options below. Each option can be used once, more than once or not at all.

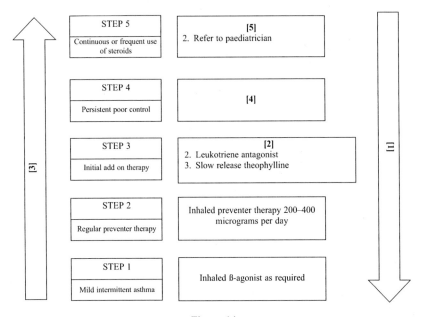

Figure 14

A. Montelukast 10 mg nocte
B. Salbutamol 100 micrograms
C. Nebulised Ipratropium bromide
D. Low-dose Prednisolone
E. Inhaled Salmeterol +/- Beclomethasone 400 micrograms
F. Step up to remove symptoms
G. Beclomethasone 800 micrograms
H. Reduced aerobic exercise
I. Doxycycline
J. Increased peak flow measurements
K. Step-down to find and maintain lowest controlling step

38. Blank 1
39. Blank 2
40. Blank 3
41. Blank 4
42. Blank 5

Neurological problems – Balance problems

43. You recently referred a 32 year old woman to the ophthalmology on-call for painful loss of vision in her right eye. Ophthalmology then referred her to a neurologist as on detailed history taking, she revealed that she has been having brief episodes of slurred speech and problems with balance for the last 1-2 years. See Figure 15 which is a copy of the MRI brain scan report which the neurologists had organised for the patient:

MRI Brain report

Multiple foci of high T2 signal density seen within the periventricular white matter of both cerebral hemispheres and the spinal cord (? plaques).

These may be suggestive of a demyelinating process.

Figure 15

A lumbar puncture was also performed, which showed oligoclonal bands and a slightly raised level of CSF protein.

Select the **SINGLE MOST** likely diagnosis? Select **ONE** option only.

A. Myasthenia gravis
B. Multiple sclerosis
C. Muscular dystrophy
D. Acute disseminated encephalomyelitis
E. Brain tumour

Skin problems – Rash

44. A 25 year old obese woman has a 2 day history of increasing lethargy, neck stiffness and vomiting. She noticed a few small spots develop on her leg today and her mother brought her in to see you immediately. She is pyrexial at 38.3 °C and is Kernig positive. You also notice a non-blanching, purpuric rash on her right leg (see Figure 16 below).

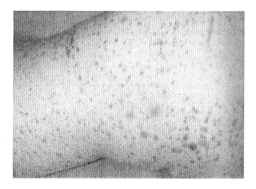

Figure 16

What is the **SINGLE MOST** likely diagnosis? Select **ONE** option only.

A. Cellulitis
B. Meningococcal septicaemia
C. Chickenpox
D. Measles
E. Anaphylaxis

Clinical governance – Audit questions 45–49

See the audit cycle shown in Figure 17 below and fill in the missing boxes from the options below. Select **ONE** option only.

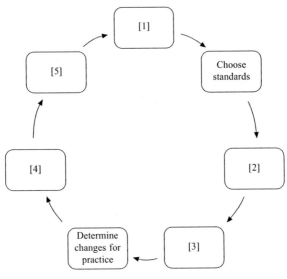

Figure 17

A. Decide topic
B. Choose criteria
C. Re-audit
D. Stop data collection
E. Implement changes
F. Collect data
G. Analyse data
H. Choose new standards

45. Blank 1
46. Blank 2
47. Blank 3
48. Blank 4
49. Blank 5

Neurological problems – Facial weakness

50. One of your GP colleagues recently diagnosed a patient with Horner's syndrome, based on the signs shown in Figure 18 below. Which set of symptoms do you think the patient presented with? Select **ONE** option only.

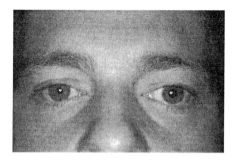

Figure 18

A. Mydriasis + partial ptosis + anhydrosis
B. Miosis + partial ptosis + anhydrosis
C. Mydriasis + enopthalmos
D. Mydriasis + partial ptosis + enopthalmos
E. Miosis + exophthalmos

Eye problems – Swelling

51.   A 62 year old man presents with severe pain and swelling around his right eye occurring and progressively worsening over the last 12–24 hours. He has a temperature of 38.4 °C, looks unwell and his right eyelids are shut due to the surrounding oedema (see Figure 19 below).

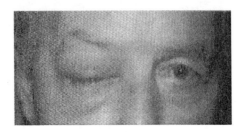

Figure 19

What is the **SINGLE MOST** appropriate next step of management? Select **ONE** option only.

A.   Trial of paracetamol and ibuprofen
B.   Send home with course of co-amoxiclav
C.   Refer routinely to a dermatologist
D.   Immediate referral to Ophthalmology for intravenous antibiotics
F.   Trial of chlorphenamine to help reduce the swelling

Drug and alcohol problems – Questions 52–56

Fill in the numbered blank spaces in Figure 20 below, using the correct answer from the options below. Each option can be used once, more than once or not at all.

STAGES OF ADDICTION

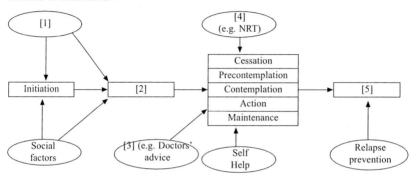

Figure 20

A. Maintenance
B. Cessation
C. Positive reinforcement
D. Beliefs
E. Conditioned response
F. Public health intervention
G. Pre-contemplation
H. Clinical intervention
I. Relapse
J. Negative reinforcement
K. Addictive Behaviour

52. Blank 1
53. Blank 2
54. Blank 3
55. Blank 4
56. Blank 5

Eye problems – Loss of vision

57. A 58 year old woman visits the surgery as she woke up this morning with painless loss of vision in her right eye. She has known hypertension and smokes 40 cigarettes per day. Fundoscopy of her right eye revealed the image shown in Figure 21 below.

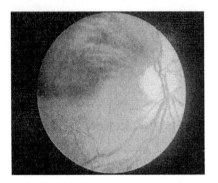

Figure 21

Select the **SINGLE MOST** likely diagnosis. Select **ONE** option only.

A. Central retinal artery occlusion
B. Retinal detachment
C. Central retinal vein occlusion
D. Glaucoma
E. Age-related macular degeneration

ENT and facial problems – Ear conditions

58. What is the most likely diagnosis of the condition shown in Figure 22? Select **ONE** option only.

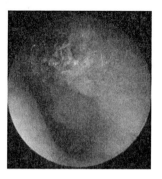

Figure 22   http://commons.wikimedia.org/wiki/Main_page

A. Otitis media
B. Otitis externa
C. Mastoiditits
D. Cholesteatoma
E. Otitis media with effusion

Evidence based practice – Chronic kidney disease questions 59–63

For Table 4 below, which is adapted from the NICE quick reference guidelines on Chronic Kidney Disease in patients with Diabetes, select the most appropriate answer from the following options below.

	eGFR greater than or = 60 eGFR 30–59	eGFR <30
ACR > 2.5 (men) or ACR > [1] (women)	Offer [2] (or [3] if intolerant) Treat blood pressure. Aim for Systolic: [4] – [5] mmHg Diastolic < 80 mmHg	Refer to specialist

Table 4

A. 3.0
B. 3.5
C. Beta blocker
D. Diuretic
E. ACE inhibitor
F. Angiotensin Receptor Blocker
G. 140
H. 130
I. 120
J. 129
K. 139
L. 149

59. Blank 1
60. Blank 2
61. Blank 3
62. Blank 4
63. Blank 5

Eye Problems – Loss of vision

64. A 74 year old man, with known atrial fibrillation, presents with an acute, persistent painless loss of vision in his left eye. He recalls that he has had episodes of transient visual loss in the same eye in the last few weeks. On examination, visual acuity is reduced to light perception in his left eye with 6/6 visual acuity in the right eye. Fundoscopy of his left eye reveals the image shown in Figure 23, which includes a pale inferior retina.

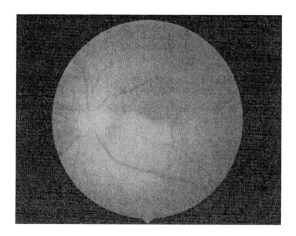

Figure 23

Select the **SINGLE MOST** likely diagnosis of his current eye problem. Select **ONE** option only.

A. Retinal vein occlusion
B. Amaurosis fugax
C. Retinal artery occlusion
D. Glaucoma
E. Age-related macular degeneration

Sexual health – Long acting reversible contraception questions 65–69

See Figure 24 adapted from the NICE quick reference guide on long acting reversible contraception below and, using the options below, select the most appropriate option to fill in the missing blanks. Each option may be used once, more than once or not at all.

Routine follow up

IUD/IUS

- At 3-[A] weeks to check threads and exclude perforation
- Return if problems or time for removal; [B]

Injectable contraceptives

- Every [C] weeks for [D], every 8 weeks for [E]

Implants

- No routine follow-up, return if problems, to change method or if time for removal

---

Figure 24

A. 4
B. 5
C. 6
D. No further follow-up needed
E. 10
F. Follow-up needed
G. 12
H. 14
I. DMPA
J. NET-EN

65. Blank 1
66. Blank 2
67. Blank 3
68. Blank 4
69. Blank 5

Skin problems – Lesion

70. A 28 year old female with a six month history of bloody diarrhoea is currently being investigated by gastroenterology. She has developed a painful lesion on her left shin which initially began as a small pustule. On examination, she now has a well-demarcated ulcer with a blue-black edge (see Figure 25).

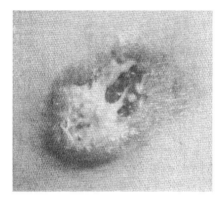

Figure 25

Select the **SINGLE MOST** likely diagnosis. Select **ONE** option only.

A. Erythema nodosum
B. Dermatitis herpetiformis
C. Pyoderma gangrenosum
D. Bullous pemphigoid
E. Leprosy

Research & academic activity – Data interpretation

71. See Figure 26 below which is a forest plot comparing Drug X with a placebo. Which of the following statements is true? Select **ONE** option only.

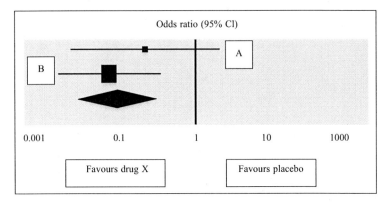

Figure 26

A. Three trials have been compared
B. Study B had a smaller sample size
C. There is a significant difference between drug X and placebo in study A
D. There is an overall significant difference between drug X and placebo
E. None of the above

ENT and facial problems – Ear conditions

72. What does the audiogram (Figure 27) below show? Select **ONE** option only.

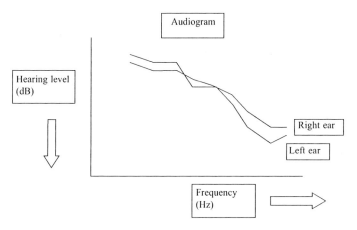

Figure 27

A. Normal hearing
B. Conductive hearing loss
C. Presbyacusis
D. Bilateral conductive deafness
E. None of the above

Eye problems – Retinal problem

73. A 36 year old male with known Acquired Immunodeficiency Syndrome (AIDS) presents with sudden visual loss. His CD4 count is now 40/mm^3. Figure 28 show the findings seen on fundoscopy.

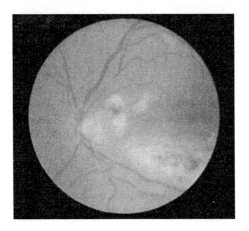

Figure 28

Select the **SINGLE MOST** appropriate diagnosis. Select **ONE** option only.

A. Retinal venous occlusion
B. Cytomegalovirus (CMV) retinitis
C. Retinal detachment
D. Age-related macular degeneration
E. Retinal tear

Management in primary care – Flu pandemic

74. See Figure 29 below regarding swine flu. Which of the following statements does

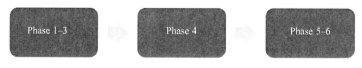

Figure 29

Phase 4 correspond to? Select **ONE** option only.

A. Animal infections, few human infections
B. Sustained human to human transmission
C. Widespread human infection in at least 2 countries
D. Pandemic
E. None of the above

ENT problems – Neck anatomy

75. Looking at Figure 30 below, what neck procedure does the incision site refer to? Select **ONE** option only.

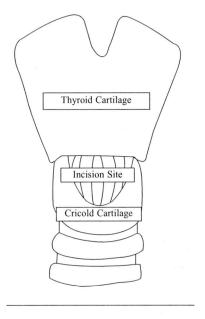

Figure 30

A. Cervical laminectomy
B. Thyroidectomy
C. Emergency airway
D. Laryngectomy
E. None of the above

Eye problems – External eye problems

76. A 70 year old man presents with sagging of both of his left lower eyelids with increased watering and irritation in both eyes (see Figure 31).

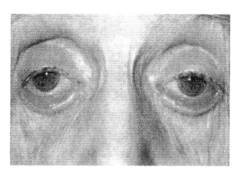

Figure 31

Select the **SINGLE MOST** likely diagnosis. Select **ONE** option only.

A. Ectropion
B. Entropion
C. External hordeolum
D. Conjunctivitis
E. Hyphaema

Metabolic problems – Bone disease

77. What disease does Figure 32 illustrate a feature of? Select **ONE** option only.

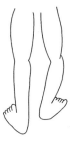

Figure 32

A. Osteoarthritis
B. Rheumatoid arthritis
C. Paget's disease of bone
D. Pseudogout
E. Gout

Respiratory problems – Peak expiratory flow rates questions 78–82

For each question below, select the correct answer from the options below. Each option can be used once, more than once or not at all.

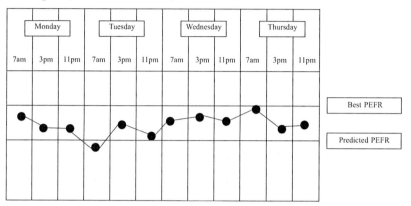

Figure 33

A. Ipratropium Bromide
B. Occupational asthma
C. Pneumothorax
D. Salbutamol
E. Emphysema
F. Anaphylaxis
G. Asthma
H. Kyphosis
I. Normal
J. Beclomethasone
K. No medication

78. What does this peak flow chart (Figure 33) demonstrate?
79. What, if anything, would you give to this patient?
80. If there was a significant difference between the peak expiratory flow rate (PEFR) at certain times of the day what would this suggest?
81. If this patient was tall and slim and suddenly became very breathless at rest what would be the most likely diagnosis?
82. If following a 30 pack year history whilst working in a chemical plant this patient's PEFR was constantly reduced what would be the most likely diagnosis?

Cardiovascular problems questions 83–87

For each question below, select the correct answer from the options below.
Each option can be used once, more than once or not at all.

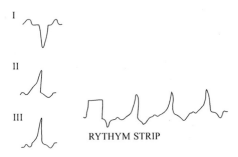

Figure 34

A. Atrial fibrillation
B. Short PR interval
C. IV Flecainide
D. Mobitz type 2
E. J wave
F. Sick sinus syndrome
G. Wolf Parkinson White
H. Paroxysmal tachycardia
I. Trifasicular block
J. Aspirin
K. Digoxin

83. What is the above rhythm shown in Figure 34?
84. What ECG changes are associated with this rhythm?
85. What condition can this rhythm lead to?
86. What is an appropriate pharmaceutical treatment for this condition?
87. What medication should never be given for this condition?

Genetics in primary care questions 88–92

You see a new patient who complains of changes to the appearance of their gums. He has rashes on his cheeks and back that he says have been there for years. You are aware that he appears to have some learning difficulties.

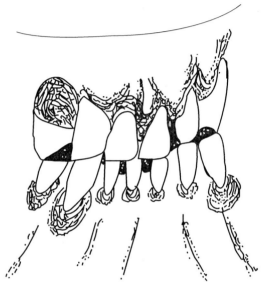

Figure 35

With regards to this history and Figure 35 above, answer the following questions using options from the list below. Each option can be used once, more than once or not at all.

A. Neurofibromatosis type I
B. Dental abscess
C. Tuberous sclerosis
D. Sex linked recessive
E. Polymorphic inheritance
F. Chemotherapy
G. Phenytoin
H. Angiofibroma
I. Skin metastases
J. Autosomal dominant
K. Gingival hyperplasia

88. What does the picture show?
89. What is the likely cause of this?
90. What is the underlying disorder?
91. What is the pattern of inheritance?
92. What is a likely diagnosis for the rash?

Respiratory problems questions 93–97

For each numbered blank space in Figure 36 below, select the correct answer from the options below. Each option can be used once, more than once or not at all.

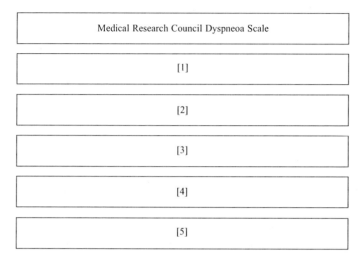

Medical Research Council Dyspneoa Scale
[1]
[2]
[3]
[4]
[5]

Figure 36

A. Too breathless to leave the house
B. Shortness of breath at rest
C. Shortness of breath when laying flat
D. Shortness of breath hurrying
E. Nocturnal wheeze most nights
F. Stops for breath after walking for a few minutes on level ground
G. Productive morning cough
H. Walks slower than contemporaries on level ground due to breathlessness
I. FEV1 <70% of predicted
J. Breathless after strenuous exercise
K. Shortness of breath at night

93. Blank 1
94. Blank 2
95. Blank 3
96. Blank 4
97. Blank 5

Women's health – Breast screening

98. Regarding Figure 37 below about breast screening what is missing box X? Select **ONE** option only.

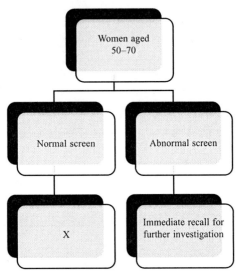

Figure 37

A. 2 yearly
B. 3 yearly
C. 4 yearly
D. 5 yearly
E. None of the above

Men's health – Penile disorders

99.   What does Figure 38 below show? Select **ONE** option only.

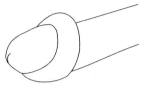

Figure 38

A.   Phimosis
B.   Paraphimosis
C.   Balanitits
D.   Inguinal-scrotal hernia
E.   None of the above

Sexual health – Missed pills

100. In Figure 39 below regarding missed pills for the combined oral contraceptive, what is the missing blank X? Select **ONE** option only.

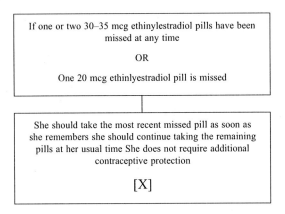

Figure 39

A. She should use emergency contraception if the missed pill was in week 1

B. She should omit the pill-free interval if the missed pill was in week 4

C. She does not require emergency contraception

D. She should use condoms for 7 days

E. None of the above

Answer section: Picture Questions

1. Blank 1 – A
2. Blank 2 – E
3. Blank 3 – H
4. Blank 4 – I
5. Blank 5 – F
6. C
   Eczema herpeticum is a severe primary herpes infection that can occur in individuals with eczema. There are widespread clusters of herpetic lesions (cold-sores and punched-out erosions). Treatment is with oral or intravenous aciclovir to treat or prevent super infection. Urgent referral to dermatology is required.

7. D
   Remember the ABCDE rule to help diagnose malignant melanoma:

   A – asymmetry   (doesn't look symmetrical)
   B – borders   (irregular border)
   C – colours   (irregular colour)
   D – diameter   (suspicious if >5 mm diameter)
   E – elevation   (raised lesions are more suspicious of malignancy)

8. E
   This is a L'Abbe plot. This is a visual representation of data comparing a treatment with a placebo. Trials in which the experimental treatment is better than the control will be in the upper left of the plot. Trials in which the control is better will be in the lower right of the plot. Trials in which the experimental and control treatment are the same will lie on the line of equality. The size of the trial is reflected in the size of the circle used.

9. C

    Oral retinoids (e.g. Roaccutane) are used only for severe acne due to their side-effects.

10. D

    This is the correct answer. Menorrhagia is the loss of more than or equal to 80ml of blood/month. A thorough history is needed assessing the amount, type and frequency of bleeding. Also associated symptoms such as pain and drug history, medical and family history of bleeding tendency needs to be elicited. Abdominal and vaginal examination is needed and then investigations required.

    NICE has guidelines on this and they say that endometrial ablation is used when there is severe impact on the quality of life and the woman has no desire to conceive, and she has a normal uterus +/– fibroids <3 cm in diameter. Dilatation and curettage is not recommended by NICE and a hysteroscopy is not used for menorrhagia.

    For more information see the NICE quick reference guide at http://www.nice.org.uk/nicemedia/pdf/CG44quickrefguide.pdf

11. B

12. F

13. E

14. K

15. C

16. E

    This is rhinophyma, which is due to severe sebaceous gland hyperplasia on the nose. Known complication of acne rosacea. More common in older men and individuals with excess alcohol intake. Long-term antibiotics (e.g. tetracycline) can be given to treat recurrences. Surgical treatment involves excision of excess soft tissue.

17. I

18. B

19. D

20. H

21. F

In short the doctor must try to reconcile their own agenda and that of their patients in order to achieve a patient-centred, effective consultation. There is an excellent article on the RCGP journal for associates in training, (InnovAirt Vol 2, Issue 2, Feb 2009) concerning the consultation process. This article is easy to read and contains descriptions of the essential consultation models; and illustrates the altering thoughts of the doctor and their patient during the consultation.

22. C

This is a positively skewed distribution with the tail of the graph being in the positive direction. In this kind of distribution the mode < median < mean. The opposite is true in a negatively skewed distribution. In a normal distribution, the mean = median = mode.

23. C

This is acne rosacea. Acne rosacea can be treated with topical metronidazole gel (first-line) or oral antibiotics (e.g. tetracycline) if not responding, or if extensive papules/pustules. Complications of acne rosacea are: rhinophyma.

24. G

25. I

26. K

27. D

28. F

29. B

Non-alcoholic steatosis (fatty liver) is associated with truncal obesity. GGT is usually raised and AST:ALT ratio is typically <1 (if >1, then fibrosis is more likely). May progress to cirrhosis, but liver failure is uncommon. Many patients will develop impaired glucose tolerance or diabetes later in life.

30. D

NICE guidance on referral for suspected cancer (2005) suggests that urgent referral is required for any non-menstruating woman with unexplained iron deficiency anaemia and a haemoglobin <10.0 g/dL.

31. Blank 1 – A

32. Blank 2 – C

33. Blank 3 – D

34. Blank 4 – F

35. Blank 5 – B
    In women of reproductive age the most common cause of vaginal discharge is physiological. Other causes include:

    - Bacterial vaginosis and Candida (non – sexually transmitted)
    - Trichomonas vaginalis, Chlamydia trachomatis and Neisseria gonorrhoea (sexually transmitted)
    - Foreign body, cervical polyps and ectopy, fistulae, genital tract malignancy, allergic reactions (non-infective)

    See the Faculty of Sexual and Reproductive Health guidance on http://www.ffprhc.org.uk/admin/uploads/326_VaginalDischargeGuidance.pdf for more information.

36. E
    Guttate psoriasis can occur after an episode of acute pharyngitis (Group B haemolytic streptococcus) in those who are predisposed to developing psoriasis. The majority of patients have an acute self-limiting illness (especially in children), but some may then subsequently develop chronic psoriasis. The lesions look like salmon pink, dew drop papules mainly on the trunk, but they may also appear on the head and limbs.

37. E
    This is Bell's palsy. The ear pain may suggest Ramsay-Hunt syndrome, but ENT examination is normal and ear pain is quite common in Bell's palsy.

    Bell's palsy is an acute, unilateral facial paralysis of which the cause is unknown, even though herpes simplex virus has been implicated. It is a lower motor neurone lesion, so the forehead is affected (forehead is spared in upper motor neurone lesions as it is bilaterally innervated).

    Within 72 hours of onset of Bell's palsy, it is recommended that prednisolone 25 mg is given twice daily for 10 days. Giving acyclovir has no proven benefit.

    Reference: Sullivan F. et al. Early treatment with prednisolone or acyclovir in Bell's palsy. N Engl J Med 2007; 357:1598

38. Blank 1 – K

39. Blank 2 – E

40. Blank 3 – F

41. Blank 4 – G

42. Blank 5 – D

43. B

This lady has multiple sclerosis which is an autoimmune process characterised by repeated episodes of inflammation in the brain and spinal cord, resulting in demyelination. This manifests as neurological symptoms which are disseminated in space and time.

Types of multiple sclerosis:

Relapsing/remitting MS	Symptoms come and go
Secondary progressive MS	Follows on from relapsing/remitting MS – symptoms get worse, with few remissions
Primary progressive MS	Symptoms worsen from the beginning

Presenting Symptoms:
Painful loss of vision (optic neuritis) double vision, nystagmus.
Intermittent dysarthria, ataxia, paraesthesia
Urinary/faecal incontinence

44. B

This is meningococcal septicaemia and should not be missed!

45. Box 1 – A

46. Box 2 – F

47. Box 3 – G

48. Box 4 – E

49. Box 5 – C

Audits are a key part of clinical governance. The steps are self explanatory and in order to close the audit cycle a re-audit is needed to check that the implemented changes have had an effect.

50. B

Horner's syndrome is characterised by: slight ptosis, miosis (small pupil), anhydrosis (loss of sweating on one side) and enopthalmos (sunken eye).

Anhydrosis of face, arm, trunk – central lesion: causes include stroke, MS, syringomyelia, tumour, encephalitis

Anhydrosis of face – pre-ganglionic lesion: causes include Pancoast's tumour, thyroidectomy, trauma, cervical rib

No anhydrosis – post-ganglionic lesion: causes include carotid artery dissection, carotid aneurysm, cavernous sinus thrombosis, cluster headache

51. D

This is orbital cellulitis – an ophthalological emergency, which may need involvement from ENT team too.

52. D

53. A

54. F – Giving health advice is a public health intervention

55. H – Prescribing treatment for particular patients is a clinic intervention

56. I

This model was adapted from that in Jane Ogden's *Health Psychology: A Textbook* (2nd Edition, Jane Ogden.) It is important to recognize the stages of addiction and whereabouts in this cycle your patient lies. For example, understanding that a patient is in the pre-contemplative position can help you to understand why he or she may not be enthused by your offers of help.

57. C

This is central retinal vein occlusion. Characterised by haemorrhages throughout the fundus (blood-storm pattern) with cotton wool spots. Visual loss is related to degree of macular involvement. Requires immediate referral to on-call ophthalmologist.

58. D

This is a cholesteatoma. A cholesteatoma is stratified squamous epithelium that invades the middle ear. The cause is not known. It can cause a foul smelling discharge and deafness. It also is associated with vertigo, facial nerve palsy, cerebral abscess formation and cerebellopontine angle syndrome. On otoscopy an attic crust is seen in the uppermost part of the ear drum. Refer to ENT as surgery may be needed to remove the invasive tissue.

59. Blank 1 – B

60. Blank 2 – E

61. Blank 3 – F

62. Blank 4 – I

63. Blank 5 – J

Chronic kidney disease is based on eGFR, stage 1 eGFR > 90 is normal. There are 5 stages. Albumin creatinine ratio (ACR) should be used in preference to identify proteinuria as it has a greater sensitivity. ACE inhibitors/ARBs should be offered to all non-diabetic people with CKD and ACR greater than or = 30 mg/mmol. In diabetics microalbuminuria (ACR >2.5 mg/mmol in men and >3.5 mg/mmol in women is clinically significant. If the eGFR is also > 30 then diabetics should be offered an ACE inhibitor or ARB. The blood pressure target should be 120–129 mmHg systolic

and <80 mmgHg diastolic. If the eGFR <30 then you should refer to a specialist.

People with the following risk factors should be offered testing for CKD:

- Diabetes
- Hypertension
- Cardiovascular disease
- Structural renal tract disease, renal calculi or prostatic hypertrophy
- Family history of CKG stage 5 or hereditary kidney disease
- Opportunistic detection of proteinuria or haematuria

For more information see the NICE quick reference guide at http://www.nice.org.uk/nicemedia/pdf/CG073QuickRefGuide.pdf

64. C
This is central retinal artery occlusion. It is most commonly associated with atrial fibrillation and valvular heart disease. In 90% of cases, visual acuity ranges from light perception to counting fingers only. There may have been earlier episodes of transient visual loss (amaurosis fugax), which this patient had. Fundoscopy reveals a pale retina and a 'cherry-red spot' at the fovea (choroid/ retinal pigment seen through very thin overlying foveola retina). This requires immediate referral to the on-call ophthalmologist.

65. Blank A – C

66. Blank B – D

67. Blank C – G

68. Blank D – I

69. Blank E – J
The Long Acting Reversible Contraceptives (IUD, IUS, injectables and implants) are all more cost effective than the combined oral contraceptive pill even at 1 year of use.

Copper IUDs are licensed for 5–10 years depending on the type. In insertion is at the age of 40 or above they can be left in until contraception is no longer needed. IUS is licensed for 5 years and if the woman is 45 years or older at time of insertion, and she is not having periods with the IUS in place, then it can be left in until contraception is no longer needed. Both the IUD and IUS have an expulsion rate of 1 in 20, ectopic pregnancy rate of 1 in 20 if she does become pregnant and a uterine perforation rate of less than 1 in 1000.

IUDs and IUSs should have a check at 3–6 weeks to make sure the strings can be felt and to exclude perforation. Injectables include DMPA, given 12 weekly and NET-EN given 8 weekly. Implants last for 3 years and do not require any routine follow up once fitted.

For more information see the NICE quick reference guide at http://www.nice.org.uk/nicemedia/pdf/cg030quickrefguide.pdf

70. C

Pyoderma gangrenosum is associated with inflammatory bowel disease, rheumatoid arthritis, liver disease and multiple myeloma. It often starts as a small red pustule which then turns into a deep, painful, ulcer which has a well-defined blue-violet margin. It occurs mainly on the legs.

71. D

There is a significant result for clinical failure as the summary result does not cross the midline.

This is a forest plot showing the results of the 2 trials. The size of the trial is reflected by the size of the square used. The diamond is the summary result of the trials and in this case as it does not cross the midline it is a significant result which favours the drug X compared to placebo. If the midline is crossed then there is no significant effect.

72. C

This shows the high frequency loss of presbyacusis. This is bilateral sensorineural hearing loss that occurs in the elderly. It is gradual in onset and due to high frequency loss. A hearing test will determine this and a hearing aid may be needed.

73. B

Cytomegalovirus (CMV) retinitis occurs in those who are immunocompromised, especially as an opportunistic infection in Acquired Immunodeficiency Syndrome (AIDS), when the CD4 count becomes low. May be asymptomatic or present with sudden visual loss (untreatable). Features: 'pizza pie' fundus – retinal spots (small retinal infarctions) and flame-shaped haemorrhages.

74. B

This is stage 4. The WHO declared Swine flu as phase 6 pandemic phase on 11 June 2009. Human cases of swine flu (H1N1) were first identified in Mexico. It is a novel influenza A virus. It produces influenza type symptoms. The virus is sensitive to oseltamivir and zanamivir. See the Health Protection Agency website for more information on Swine Flu on www.hpa.org.uk. Also see the World Health Organisation website on www.who.int/en/

75. C
This is the location of an emergency airway. Be aware of the structures in the neck and also make sure you know about acute emergencies.

76. A
Ectropion is the eversion of the lower eyelids and eyelashes with subsequent pooling of the tears and dryness/irritation of the eye. Most common cause is old age with natural loss of muscle tone and orbital fat.

77. C
Paget's disease involves disorganised and excessive bone formation and resorption. Symptoms include pain, aggravated by weight bearing. Patients can get bowing of the legs, frontal bossing of the forehead. Alkaline phosphatise is high, calcium and phosphate are normal. Treatment involves pain relief and bisphosphonates. Complications include pathological fractures, high output CCF and deafness and bone sarcoma.

78. I

79. K

80. G

81. C

82. E

83. G – WPW syndrome as it has a short PR interval, upward sloping delta wave and wide QRS.

84. B

85. H

86. C – disopyramide or a beta-blocker can also be used

87. K – drugs like digoxin and verapamil block the atrioventricular node. They increase conduction via the accessory pathway leading to sustained tachycardia.

88. K

89. G – Gingival hyperplasia is a side effect of certain medication such as Phenytoin, an old anti-epileptic drug.

90. C – Tuberous sclerosis is a genetic disorder that affects most organ systems due to the formation of hamartia (malformed tissue), hamartomas (benign tumour growth) and rarely hamartoblastomas.

91. J

92. H – the angiofibromas (adenoma sebaceum) are hamartomas.

93. J

94. D

95. H

96. F

97. A
It is now part of the quality outcomes framework for each patient with COPD to have their MRC grade documented.

98. B
Within the national breast screening scheme, women above 50 have a mammogram three yearly. In women over 50 the screening program has reduced the mortality from breast cancer by at least 25%. See the national screening website for more information on www.cancerscreening.nhs.uk

99. B
Paraphimosis is when the foreskin cannot be pulled back after retraction. Oedema develops and pain can result. Treatment involves manual reduction using ice packs and local anaesthetic jelly as a lubricant and also for pain relief. If this fails the patient should be admitted for surgery.

Phimosis is the inability to retract the foreskin. Presentation is with poor urine stream, recurrent balanitis, pain on intercourse in adults. Treatment is with circumcision.

100. C
She does not require emergency contraception.

For more information see the Faculty of Sexual and Reproductive Health guidance at http://www.ffprhc.org.uk/admin/uploads/MissedPillRules%20.pdf

Mock Paper: 200 Questions

Cardiovascular problems – Hypertension

1. A 59 year old woman with hypertension on bendroflumethiazide
    2.5 mg od, amlodipine 10 mg od and ramipril 2.5 mg od presents
    with pitting ankle oedma.

    What is the **SINGLE MOST** appropriate next step in management?
    Select **ONE** option only.

    A. Stop bendroflumethiazide
    B. Stop amlodipine
    C. Stop ramipril
    D. Increase dose of bendroflumethiazide
    E. Add-in furosemide

Cardiovascular problems – Heart failure

2. Which one of the following should be avoided in the management
    of heart failure?

    Select **ONE** option only.

    A. Ramipril
    B. Digoxin
    C. Carvedilol
    D. Nifedipine
    E. Spironolactone

Neurological problems – Stroke

3. Which of the following is **NOT** usually a feature of an ischaemic stroke (as opposed to a haemorrhagic one)?

    Select **ONE** option only.

    A. CT brain is usually normal or only shows subtle changes
    B. Up to a third of patients will often have a preceding TIA
    C. Hypertension is often present
    D. Signs of raised intracranial pressure are often absent in early stages
    E. Usually occur with activity

Neurological problems – Dementia

4. You refer one of your patients to the Memory Clinic. You perform a routine dementia blood screen which comes back normal.

    Which one of the following statements is correct about the use of neuroimaging in diagnosing dementia? Select **ONE** option only.

    A. Neuroimaging is only required if focal neurology detected on examination
    B. Neuroimaging is required for all patients < 70 years old
    C. Neuroimaging is required for all patients > 80 years old
    D. Neuroimaging is required for all patients
    E. Neuroimaging is only required if examination reveals cardiovascular abnormality (e.g. carotid bruit, atrial fibrillation, etc.)

Patient safety – Fitness to fly

A. Can not fly
B. No restriction
C. 24 hours
D. 48 hours
E. 7 days
F. 10 days
G. 4 weeks
H. 6 weeks
I. 5 days
J. 14 days

For each of the following cases below select the **SINGLE MOST** appropriate flying restriction from the options above. Each option may be used once, more than once or not at all.

  5. Colonoscopy
  6. Fracture and 10hr flight
  7. Percutaneous coronary intervention
  8. Pneumothorax
  9. Anaemia with a haemoglobin level of 10g/dL

Care of older adults – Falls

  10. According to NICE guidance (2004) of assessment and prevention of falls, which of the following is **NOT** a risk factor for falls?

  Select **ONE** option only.

  A. Increasing age
  B. Cognitive impairment
  C. Multiple previous falls
  D. Visual impairment
  E. Upper limb weakness/arthritis

Skin problems – Eczema

11. Which of the following is the most potent steroid cream?

    Select **ONE** answer only.

    A. Hydrocortisone 1%
    B. Dermovate
    C. Betnovate RD
    D. Betnovate
    E. Eumovate

Care of people with cancer and palliative care – Referral for suspected cancer

12. Which of the following patients does **NOT** meet the criteria for urgent referral to colorectal services within 2 weeks?

    Select **ONE** option only.

    A. A 70 year old man with new onset of constipation for the last 3 months
    B. A 37 year old male with a palpable rectal mass
    C. A 50 year old woman with diarrhoea and rectal bleeding for the last 8 weeks
    D. A 55 year old woman with unexplained iron deficiency anaemia
    E. A 64 year old man with rectal bleeding for the last 3 months

Teaching, mentoring and clinical supervision – Learning theory

13. Which of the following is **NOT** a feature of the cognitive theory of learning?

    Select **ONE** option only.

    A. New information learned is shaped to fit with the learner's existing knowledge
    B. People learn by repeating things in different situations and by getting rewarded
    C. Existing information is modified to accommodate the new information learned.
    D. People learn by organising information and mentally giving it some structure
    E. People learn by receiving feedback from other people

Neurological problems – Migraines

14. Which of the following is **NOT** used in the prevention of migraines?

    Select **ONE** option only.

    A. Atenolol
    B. Amitriptyline
    C. Sumatriptan
    D. Sodium valproate
    E. Topiramate

Skin problems – Skin lesions

15. A 53 year old obese woman, with known poorly controlled diabetes and heavy smoker, has noticed she has developed some yellow lumps around her eyelids. On examination, she has yellow flat plaques on the medial aspects of her eyelids (see Figure 40).

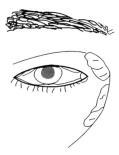

Figure 40

What is the **SINGLE MOST** likely diagnosis? Select **ONE** option only.

A. Milia
B. Syringoma
C. Psoriasis
D. Basal cell carcinoma
E. Xanthelasma

Neurological problem – Peripheral nerve lesion

16. A 30 year old man had several alcoholic drinks last Saturday night
    and was found by his girlfriend the morning after with his right
    arm draped over a chair. On examination, his right wrist remains
    flexed and he is unable to extend it. There is also some sensory
    loss on the back of his right hand near the base of his thumb.

    Which nerve correlates to these signs and symptoms? Select **ONE**
    option only.

    A. Median nerve
    B. Ulnar nerve
    C. Radial nerve
    D. Sciatic nerve
    E. Femoral nerve

ENT and facial problems – Neck lumps

A. Lymph node
B. Lymphoma
C. Cystic hygroma
D. Branchial cyst
E. Goitre
F. Pharyngeal pouch
G. Thyroglossal cyst
H. Carotid aneurysm
I. Cervical rib

For each of the cases below select the **SINGLE MOST** appropriate
diagnosis from the options above. Each option may be used once, more
than once or not at all.

17. A young man presents with a midline swelling which moves
    upwards on protrusion of the tongue
18. A woman presents with a mass on her right side of the neck which
    is pulsatile
19. A man presents with a left sided swelling after having had an upper
    respiratory tract infection. It is a smooth swelling.
20. A man presents with dysphagia, cough and regurgitation. On
    examination he has a midline lump which gargles on palpation.
21. A woman has been having night sweats and weight loss. She has
    a rubbery feeling swelling on the left side of her neck which is
    not tender.

Neurological problems – Peripheral nerve lesion

22. A 32 year old woman, who loves wearing tight-fitting boots for prolonged periods of time, has recently developed pain around her ankles and toes in her left lower leg. Symptoms are worst at night and are reproducible when you repeatedly tap the nerve behind her left ankle.

    Which nerve correlates to these signs and symptoms? Select **ONE** option only.

    A. Tibial nerve
    B. Common peroneal nerve
    C. Sciatic nerve
    D. Femoral nerve
    E. Ulnar nerve

Genetics in primary care – Down's syndrome

23. Which of the following features is **NOT** associated with Down's syndrome?

    Select **ONE** option only.

    A. Epicanthic folds
    B. Cataracts
    C. Brushfield spots (white dots) on the iris
    D. Increased prevalence of keratoconus
    E. Kayser-Fleischer rings (darkish pigmented ring at outer margin of cornea)

Patient safety – Organisations

24. Which one of the following organisations does **NOT** deal directly with patient safety?

    Select the **SINGLE MOST** appropriate organisation. Select **ONE** option only.

    A. British Medical Association (BMA)
    B. General Medical Council (GMC)
    C. Medicine and Healthcare products Regulatory Agency (MHRA)
    D. Health and Safety executive (HSE)
    E. National Patient Safety Agency (NPSA)

Promoting equality and valuing diversity – Discrimination

25. Regarding the prevention of discrimination against disabled doctors which of the actions below could be expected of a GP practice?

    Select the **SINGLE MOST** appropriate action. Select **ONE** option only.

    A. Give extra weighting to GP vacancy applicants who have significant disability
    B. Spend £13,000 pounds installing a wheel chair ramp so that the disabled salaried GP can get into his room in his wheel chair instead of having to use his crutches.
    C Arrange a weekly practice meeting to allow the dyslexic salaried GP to discuss any problems he's been having with the entire practice staff.
    D Pay for private counseling sessions for a GP partner with a long history of mental illness
    E. Provide a fully converted car for a profoundly disabled doctor for personal and work use.

Respiratory problems – Peak expiratory flow rates

A. Ipratropium Bromide
B. Pulmonary Rehabilitation
C. Pneumothorax
D. Salbutamol
E. Emphysema
F. Anaphylaxis
G. Asthma
H. Kyphosis
I. Normal
J. Beclomethasone
K. No medication

For each question below, select the **SINGLE MOST** appropriate option from the list above. Each option can be used once, more than once or not at all.

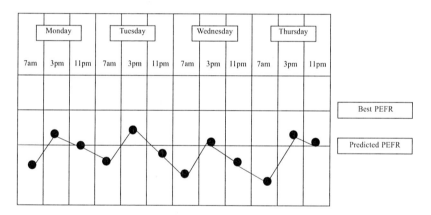

Figure 41

26. What does this peak flow chart demonstrate?
27. What, if anything, would you give to this patient if he complained of breathlessness?
28. If there was a significant difference between the peak expiratory flow rate (PEFR) at certain times of the day what would this suggest?
29. If the patient suddenly became very breathless at rest what would the most likely diagnosis be?
30. What would you offer this patient if he complained that his symptoms were having a disabling effect on his life?

Healthy people: Promoting health and preventing disease

31. Regarding the quality of a screening test which of the following statements are **TRUE**?

    Select the **SINGLE MOST** appropriate response. Select **ONE** option only.

    A. The False Positive: False Negative ratio must be more than 1.5
    B. There must be an effective treatment at least 5 years post diagnosis
    C. There must be an adequate target patient participation
    D. Screening intervals are dependent on the patient's age and co-morbidites
    E. The patient must be motivated enough to follow up the screening results.

Care of acutely ill people – Chest pain

32. A 25 year old patient presents to your GP clinic at 9 am on a Saturday morning. He was on his stag-do last night and today complains of a gnawing central chest pain that has been there since 7 am this morning. He is clutching his chest. He is breathless when he tells you this but is also quite anxious. He has a history of asthma as a child and was last treated for anxiety.

    Select the **SINGLE MOST** appropriate management step. Select **ONE** option only.

    A. Give him nebulized Salbuatmol
    B. Send him for an urgent Xray on Monday morning
    C. Give him Aspirin 300 mg
    D. Refer him for an urgent appointment with a Community Psychiatric Nurse
    E. Give him Omeprazole 40 mg and ask him to return in one month

Promoting equality and valuing diversity – Benefits

A. Disability living allowance
B. Attendance allowance
C. Income support
D. Job seekers allowance
E. Statutory sick pay
F. Bereavement allowance
G. State pension
H. No benefits claimable
I. Carers allowance

For each of the cases below select the **SINGLE MOST** appropriate benefit from options above. Each option may be used once, more than once or not at all.

33. Payment to a 47 year old woman whose husband has passed away recently

34. A 64 year old man who has a physical disability for which he needs help caring for himself and has difficulty walking

35. A woman who has recently started a job with a bank under a contract of service has become sick and has been off now for 5 days.

36. A 66 year old woman with a physical disability for which she needs help with self caring.

37. A 32 year old man who is the main carer for his mum who has dementia

Genetics in primary care – general facts

38.   As a GP Registrar you are required to have a general knowledge of genetic disease. With regards to this fact which of these statements is **TRUE**?

Select the **SINGLE MOST** appropriate response. Select **ONE** option only.

A.   A MINIMUM of one in ten consultations will be due to a disorder/disease with a genetic element.
B.   All genetic disease must be referred to a clinical geneticist
C.   It is your duty to offer termination of pregnancy to any woman at risk of delivering a baby with a genetic disorder
D.   Most illnesses with a genetic component are rare
E.   Genetic disease counseling must be available in every practice

Metabolic problems – Microalbuminaemia

39.   An 18 year old woman who is currently on the depot injection for contraception presents having recently been diagnosed with diabetes Type1. She has started insulin therapy but during a recent review in the diabetes clinic she was found to have microalbuminuria and no signs of infection. Her observations are normal (Temp 36.9 C, HR 76, BP 113/80). What is the most appropriate next step?

Select **ONE** option only.

A.   Offer a pregnancy test
B.   Offer Co-Amoxiclav
C.   Offer Ramipril
D.   Offer Co-Amoxiclav after ruling out pregnancy.
E.   Offer a diuretic

ENT and facial problems – Ear conditions

40. A 6 year old boy has been having pain in his right ear and been unwell with a cold the last few days. On otoscopy you see the ear as seen in Figure 42. What condition does Figure 42 illustrate? Select **ONE** option only.

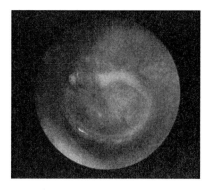

Figure 42

A. Otitis externa
B. Otitis media
C. Otitis media with effusion
D. Normal ear
E. Otosclerosis

Respiratory problems – COPD

41. You see a 60 year old postman with COPD who is on salbutamol, atrovent and a mucolytic. He complains of persistent shortness of breath despite this therapy. What is the most appropriate next step?

Select **ONE** option only.

A. Rotating antibiotics: Augmentin/Doxycycline/Clarithromycin
B. Prednisolone 30 mg po for 7 days
C. Pulmonary rehabilitation
D. 4 week trail of inhaled Beclomethasone
E. Oral Aminophylline

Respiratory problems – shortness of breath

42. An 84 year old Polish man presents to your clinic with a four week history of cough and shortness of breath. He denies any other systemic symptoms. He has always smoked 10 cigarettes a day since his days as a prisoner of war in the 1940's. He has recently visited a friend who is a keen bird fancier.

    Select the **SINGLE MOST** likely diagnosis? Select **ONE** option only.

    A. Extrinsic Allergic Alveolitis
    B. Tuberculosis
    C. Bronchial Carcinoma
    D. Pulmonary Fibrosis
    E. Pulmonary Embolism

Care of people with mental health problems – Mental health sections

A. Section 2
B. Section 3
C. Section 4
D. Section 5(2)
E. Section 5(4)
F. Section 117
G. Section 135
H. Section 136
I. Section 12

For each of the cases below select the **SINGLE MOST** appropriate section from the options above. Each option may be used once, more than once or not at all.

43. Allows someone to be detained for assessment for 28 days
44. Nurse's holding power which lasts six hours. This allows urgent detention of a patient who is already under hospital treatment
45. Doctor's holding power which lasts 72 hours
46. Allows admission for treatment lasting 6 months
47. Enables the police to transfer a person suffering from a mental illness from a public place to a place of safety for assessment

Respiratory problems – COPD

48. A 60 year old patient with COPD presents to your clinic very distressed. For the past year her symptoms, especially breathlessness, have become progressively worse. She complains that her symptoms have rendered her disabled and unable to function normally. At a recent respiratory clinic her capillary blood gas results were: pH 7.36, pCO_2 5.90kPa, pO_2 8.0kPa, BE – 2.3. She is currently taking Salbutamol 5mg nebulised QDS, Ipratropium Bromide 18 micrograms OD and Beclomethasone 800micrograms bd. She states that she wants you to help to end her life.

Select the **SINGLE MOST** appropriate option below. Select **ONE** option only.

A. Offer oxygen as required and a vial of potassium chloride for self use

B. Offer Prednisolone 30mg OD for 10 days, counselling and antidepressants

C. Offer long-term oxygen therapy, counselling and antidepressants

D. Offer pulmonary rehabilitation, counselling and antidepressants

E. Offer short burst oxygen for the relief of symptoms, counselling and antidepressants

Metabolic problems – Obesity

49. You have been helping an obese 50 year old woman with weight loss with little success. Which of these interventions is least helpful in weight management?

Select **ONE** option only.

A. Orlisat

B. Healthy eating advice

C. Exercise

D. Group therapy

E. Low calorie diet

Rheumatology/Musculoskeletal system – Hip problems

50. An elderly woman has had a fall and is now complaining of right hip pain and is walking with a limp. On examination her right leg is externally rotated.

Select the **SINGLE MOST** appropriate diagnosis from the options below. Select **ONE** option only.

A. Fractured neck of femur
B. Septic arthritis
C. Osteoarthritis
D. Hip dislocation
E. None of the above

Research and academic activity – Statistical values

	Disease positive	Disease negative
Test positive	A	B
Test negative	C	D

Table 5

Using the above table select the **SINGLE MOST** appropriate answer from the options below which describes the following terms. Each option may be used once, more than once or not at all.

A. A/A+C
B. D/B+D
C. A/A+B
D. D/C+D
E. A+C/B+D
F. B/A+B
G. C/C+D
H. A/A+B+C+D

51. Sensitivity
52. Specificity
53. Positive predictive value
54. Negative predictive value

Research and academic activity – Calculating results

1, 2, 2, 3, 3, 3, 5, 6, 6, 7, 8

From the set of numbers above, select the **SINGLE MOST** appropriate answer from the options below for the following questions. Each option may be used once, more than once or not at all.

A. 1
B. 2
C. 3
D. 4
E. 6
F. 7
G. 8
H. 9
I. 10

55. What is the mode?
56. What is the median?
57. What is the mean?
58. What is the range?

Rheumatology/Musculoskeletal system – Shoulder problems

59. An elderly man presents with pain which has got progressively worse over the last few months. He now has restricted movement of his left shoulder in all directions.

    Select the **SINGLE MOST** appropriate answer from the options below. Select **ONE** option only.

    A. Ruptured long head of biceps
    B. Shoulder dislocation
    C. Adhesive capsulitis
    D. Rotator cuff injury
    E. Acromioclavicular joint problem

Metabolic problems – Jaundice

60. A 24 year old man complains of going 'a little yellow every now and again'. He says this problem started soon after he was born. He was fine until the last 2 years when he noticed he looked yellow only when he fell ill (e.g. sore throat), but otherwise has no symptoms. On examination, he appears mildly jaundiced but abdominal examination is unremarkable. You refer him for fasting liver function tests which show the following results:

Bilirubin	62 μmol/L	(0 – 17 μmol/L)
Alkaline Phosphatase (ALP)	150 u/L	(100 – 300 u/L)
Aspartate Transaminase (AST)	32 iu/L	(5 – 42 iu/L)
Alanine Transaminase (ALT)	30 iu/L	(5 – 42 iu/L)
Gamma Gluteryl Transaminase (GGT)	9 iu/L	(5 – 30 iu/L)

Table 6

Which is the **SINGLE MOST** likely diagnosis? Select **ONE** option only.

A. Viral hepatitis
B. Gall stones
C. Pancreatitis
D. Crigler-Najjar syndrome
E. Gilbert's syndrome

Management in primary care – Practice based commissioning

61. According to the new Practice based commissioning budget guidance from 2009/2010, which of the following is **NOT** a weighted component of the PBC budget?

Select **ONE** option only.

A. Acute
B. Maternity
C. Prescribing
D. Mental health
E. Children

Research and academic activity – Statistics

62. A study was done looking at a new drug (Drug B) compared with a placebo in improving symptoms of Irritable Bowel Syndrome. Using the data in the table below, what is the odds ratio of a patient having improvement in symptoms using drug B compared to a patient taking placebo? Select **ONE** option only.

	Number of patients	Improvement in symptoms
Drug B	100	70
Placebo	80	20

Table 7

   A. 0.3
   B. 3
   C. 4
   D. 7
   E. None of the above

Neurological problems – Dementia

63. According to the NICE guidance on dementia, which of the following investigations is **NOT** routinely required when investigating suspected dementia?

Select **ONE** option only.

   A. Thyroid function tests
   B. B12 and folate
   C. Glucose
   D. Full blood count
   E. Syphilis serology

Rheumatology/Musculoskeletal system – Management of knee arthritis

64. Which of the following symptoms is the only reason for referral for arthroscopic lavage and debridement of the knee?

Select **ONE** option only.

A. Pain
B. Stiffness
C. Reduced function
D. Giving way
E. Locking

Patient safety – DVLA

65. According to the Drivers Vehicle Licensing Agency (DVLA) which one of the following does **NOT** require you to stop driving?

Select **ONE** option only.

A. Coronary angioplasty 2 days ago
B. Epileptic whose last seizure was 10 months ago
C. Simple faint
D. MI 3 weeks ago
E. Pacemaker insertion 4 days ago

Evidence based practice – Management of urinary incontinence

66. According to the NICE 2006 Urinary Incontinence guidelines, what is the minimum recommended duration of pelvic floor muscle training for stress incontinence?

Select **ONE** option only.

A. 2 months
B. 4 months
C. 3 months
D. 1 month
E. 6 months

Sexual health – Methods of contraception

67. Which of the following statements is **NOT** true about Implanon?

    Select **ONE** option only.

    A. It is licensed for 3 years use
    B. It requires a trained professional to insert and remove it
    C. Irregular bleeding is a common adverse effect
    D. It lies subdermally
    E. It causes an increased risk of stroke

Sexual health – Antibiotic use whilst on oral contraceptives

68. A 19 year old girl taking cerazette has been prescribed a week course of antibiotics for a chest infection.

    Select the **SINGLE MOST** appropriate management from the options below. Select **ONE** option only.

    A. No need for any extra precautions
    B. Use condoms for the week she is taking the antibiotics
    C. Use condoms for the week she is taking the antibiotics and also for the following 7 days (Use condoms for a total of 14 days)
    D. Abstain from sex during the antibiotics course
    E. None of the above

Women's health – Smear test results

A. Repeat sample immediately
B. Repeat the sample in 6 months
C. Routine recall in 3 years
D. Routine recall in 5 years
E. Refer for colposcopy
F. Treat with antibiotics

For each of the following smear test results below select the **SINGLE MOST** appropriate management from the options above. Each option may be used once, more than once or not at all.

69. Clue cells present
70. Inadequate sample
71. Mild dyskaryosis
72. Severe dyskaryosis
73. A 52 year old woman with a normal smear result and previous normal smears

Men's health – Reproductive system

74. Which of the following values of a sperm count is abnormal?

    Select **ONE** option only.

    A. 60% motile
    B. 35% of normal morphology
    C. Sperm concentration 25 million/ml
    D. Volume >1ml
    E. None of the above

Care of people with cancer and palliative care – Breast cancer referral

75. Which of the following patients would you **NOT** refer urgently under the 2 week wait to the breast clinic according to NICE guidelines?

Select **ONE** option only.

A. A 45 year old man who has a unilateral, firm, subareolar mass
B. A 29 year old woman with unilateral bloody nipple discharge
C. A 37 year old woman who presents with a discrete breast lump that is present after her next period
D. A 27 year old woman with a strong family history of breast cancer
E. A 54 year old woman presents with a new breast lump. She had her menopause at the age of 51.

Sexual health – Male sterilisation

76. What is the failure rate of male sterilisation?

Select **ONE** option only.

A. 1 in 200
B. 1 in 500
C. 1 in 1000
D. 1 in 20
E. 1 in 2000

Rheumatology/Musculoskeletal system – Drug doses

77. What is the dosage of methotrexate that a patient is started on for treatment of Rheumatoid arthritis?

Select **ONE** option only.

A. 2.5mg weekly
B. 2.5mg daily
C. 7.5mg weekly
D. 5mg weekly
E. 10 mg weekly

Care of people with mental health problems – Post-traumatic stress disorder

78. Which of the following is **NOT** a feature of post-traumatic stress disorder?

    Select **ONE** option only.

    A. Nightmares
    B. Flashbacks
    C. Avoidance
    D. Obsessions
    E. Hypervigilance

Rheumatology/Musculoskeletal system – Hand, wrist and elbow problems

A. Tennis elbow
B. Golfers elbow
C. Carpal tunnel syndrome
D. Osteoarthritis
E. Ganglion
F. Trigger finger
G. Olecranon bursitis
H. De Quervain's tenosynovitis

For each of the following cases select the **SINGLE MOST** appropriate diagnosis from the options above. Each option may be used once, more than once or not at all.

79. A 66 year old woman has pain in her left wrist after doing some heavy gardening. There is pain over her radial styloid on adducting and flexing her thumb.

80. A man has pain in his right elbow which is worse on resisted pronation of the wrist.

81. A keen sportsman has pain in his elbow, worst on forced wrist extension.

82. An elderly woman has pain in her lateral 3½ digits of her left hand and she gets pins and needles in her hand which settle after she shakes her hand. On examination she has wasting of her thenar eminence.

83. A 19 year old man has come in to see you with a smooth, non-tender, firm swelling on his wrist.

Women's health – Rhesus status

84. If a pregnant women is found to be Rhesus negative, at what gestation should she be given her first anti-D injection?

Select **ONE** option only.

A. 28 weeks
B. 34 weeks
C. 20 weeks
D. 16 weeks
E. 14 weeks

Women's health – Contraindications to the combined oral contraceptive

85. Which of the following is **NOT** an absolute contraindication to using the combined contraceptive pill?

Select **ONE** option only.

A. BMI >40
B. History of stroke
C. 37 year old woman who smokes more than 15 cigarettes a day
D. Migraine with aura
E. Controlled hypertension

Management in primary care – GP contract

86. Under the General Medical Services contract, which of the following is **NOT** an additional service?

Select **ONE** option only.

A. Contraceptive services
B. Chronic disease management
C. Child health surveillance
D. Cervical screening
E. Minor surgery

Research and academic activity – Data interpretation

87. From the chart below about the number of people with a new condition X, which of the following correctly describes the results shown? Select **ONE** option only.

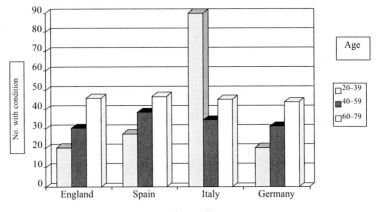

Figure 43

A. The 60–79 age group has the highest prevalence in all areas shown

B. In Italy the 20–39 group has the lowest prevalence

C. Italy has the age group with the highest prevalence

D. In England the 40–59 age group is the highest prevalence group

E. None of the above

Personal and professional responsibilities – Revalidation

88. Which of the following organisations will be in charge of revalidation?

Select **ONE** option only.

A. GMC
B. RCGP
C. BMA
D. DOH
E. MDU

Sexual health – Investigation of infertility

89. Which of the following is **NOT** regarded as an indication for the investigation of primary infertility?

Select **ONE** option only.

A. History of pelvic inflammatory disease
B. Amenorrhoea
C. Abnormal pelvic examination
D. Age 34
E. Previous pelvic organ surgery

Healthy people – Promoting health and preventing disease

A. Primary Prevention
B. The green book
C. Public Health Intervention
D. Kings Fund
E. BMA
F. Health Belief Model 1966
G. Secondary Prevention
H. Health Surveillance
I. Wilson-Junger Criteria
J. Tertiary Prevention
K. Inverse Care Law 1971

For each example below, select the **SINGLE MOST** appropriate answer from the options above. Each option can be used once, more than once or not at all.

90. A medical student at your inner city practice is researching health inequalities and wants to find information on health care policies.

91. The mother of an 18 month old baby has just returned from Pakistan and wants to know what immunisations her child needs. You are unsure as your paediatrics attachment was over a year ago.

92. A socially deprived patient attended your clinic with lethargy and weight loss. You diagnosed diabetes mellitus and started him on appropriate treatment. You have also added him onto the practice diabetes registrar which means he will have annual appointments in the diabetic clinic.

93. You have been invited by a pharmaceuticals company to pilot a new fast test for Creutzfeldt-Jakob's Disease that can be used on all patients. This test is relatively inexpensive and very accurate but you do not believe that it should be used as a screening test.

94. You see an 18 year old heterosexual man in the genitourinary medicine clinic. You give him his negative swab results but are alarmed to hear that he is still engaging in unprotected intercourse. You advise him not to, but he insists that he doesn't think he'll get HIV and even if he does, it is no longer a death sentence. He also states that his partners will not have sex with him if he wears protection therefore he thinks the benefits of not wearing protection outweigh the risks.

Women's health – Antibiotics in pregnancy

95. Regarding UTI in pregnancy, which one of the following antibiotics is most suitable?

Select **ONE** option only.

A. Ciprofloxacin
B. Augmentin
C. Doxycycline
D. Trimethoprim
E. Nitrofurantoin

Research and academic activity – Statistics

96. What is a type one error?

Select **ONE** option only

A. Rejecting the null hypothesis when it is true
B. Rejecting the null hypothesis when it is false
C. The power of the study
D. Accepting the null hypothesis when it is true
E. Accepting the null hypothesis when it is false

Clinical ethics and values based practice – Medical ethics

97. Which one of the following is **NOT** one of the four main principles of medical ethics?

Select **ONE** option only.

A. Autonomy
B. Beneficence
C. Confidentiality
D. Non-maleficence
E. Justice

Research and academic activity – Mean

98. Which one of these statements describes how to calculate the mean?

    Select **ONE** option only.

    A. Add up all the values and divide by 10
    B. Add up all the values and divide by the number of values
    C. Arrange the values from lowest to highest and it is the middle value in the list
    D. Add up all the values and multiply by the number of values
    E. None of the above

Care of children and young people – Vaccinations/ immunisations

A. Meningococcus type C (Men C) vaccine
B. Malarial Vaccine (MV)
C. Bacille Calmette-Guerin (BCG) vaccine
D. Hepatitis B vaccine
E. Pneumococcal Vaccine (PCV)
F. Measles, Mumps and Rubella (MMR) Vaccine
G. Human Papilloma Virus (HPV) vaccine
H. Diphtheria, Tetanus, Acellular Pertusis vaccine/Inactivated Polio vaccine/Haemophilus Influenzae type B (DTaP/IPV/HiB)
I. Tetanus, Diphtheria (Td)
J. Influenza vaccine
K   No vaccination necessary

For each case below, select the **SINGLE MOST** appropriate vaccination(s) from the options above. Each option can be used once, more than once or not at all.

99. The mother of a 12 year old girl has come to your clinic because the head teacher of her religious school has banned a certain vaccination. She would like her daughter to have this vaccination.

100. A 14 year old boy, who is a keen footballer but has asthma (exacerbated in the winter.) He is usually prescribed Prednisolone.

101. There has been the death of a child in the area due to an infectious illness that had previously had a very low incidence. You audit your practice records for childhood vaccinations and realise that last year a lower than normal percentage of babies around 13 months of age were vaccinated.

102. The 15 year old son of South Asian immigrants has come to your clinic requesting immunisation against vector borne infection for when he visits his grandparents. He is taking prophylactic medication but it is his first time abroad and his older brother became very unwell when he previously travelled.

103. A 2 year old boy has stepped onto a garden rake and has a serious puncture wound to his left foot. He is up-to-date with all his immunisations.

Research and academic activity – Statistics

104. In statistics, when the relative risk is greater than one, what does this mean?

     Select **ONE** option only.

     A. The intervention has no effect on the outcome being studied
     B. The intervention decreases the risk of the outcome being studied
     C. The intervention increases the risk of the outcome being studied
     D. There is no relationship between the intervention and outcome
     E. None of the above

Metabolic problems – Osteoporosis

105. Select the **SINGLE MOST** appropriate option below which describes the bone mineral density T score for osteoporosis according to the World Health Organisation?

     Select **ONE** option only.

     A. More than 0.5 standard deviations below the mean
     B. More than 1 standard deviation below the mean
     C. More than 2 standard deviations below the mean
     D. More than 2.5 standard deviations below the mean
     E. None of the above

Research and academic activity – Statistics

106. A new drug has been developed to help prevent stroke. A study was done looking at 100 patients using this new drug and 100 patients having a placebo. Over five years these patients were followed up to see the effect of the new drug. In the treatment group five patients got a stroke compared with 20 patients in the placebo group.

What is the number needed to treat? Select **ONE** option only.

A. 5
B. 6
C. 7
D. 8
E. 9

Management in primary care – Removal from practice list

107. Which of the following justifies removal from the practice list?

Select **ONE** option only.

A. Distance
B. Conflict of opinion
C. Age
D. Sex
E. Medical condition

Care of people with mental health problems – Eating disorders

108. Which of the following is used to assess eating disorders?

Select **ONE** option only.

A. CAGE
B. AUDIT
C. SCOFF
D. PAD
E. MAST

Metabolic problems – Hepatic enzyme inducers

109.   Which one of the following drugs is a liver enzyme inhibitor?

Select **ONE** option only.

A.   Carbamazepine
B.   Rifampicin
C.   Phenytoin
D.   Erythromycin
E.   Barbiturates

Evidence based practice – Clinical evidence

110.   From the list below of hierarchy of evidence, which has the least weight?

Select **ONE** option only.

A.   Cohort studies
B.   Randomised control trials
C.   Case reports
D.   Systematic reviews and meta analysis
E.   Expert opinion

Metabolic problems – Cirrhosis

A. Unknown cause
B. Alcohol
C. Wilson's disease
D. Haemochromatosis
E. Budd-Chiari syndrome
F. α_1-antitrypsin defiency
G. Primary biliary cirrhosis
H. Hepatitis C
I. Viral hepatitis
J. Autoimmune
K. Chronic Hepatitis B

For each case below, select the **SINGLE MOST** appropriate answer from the options above. Each option can be used once, more than once or not at all.

111. A 40 year old man with a history of diabetes mellitus and impotence presents with shortness of breath. Routine bloods show raised transaminases.

112. A 19 year old student presents with difficulties in concentration and low mood. The only abnormality found on examination is green-grey changes to the outside margins of his corneas. You diagnose depression. A week later he is admitted to hospital with hepatorenal failure and undergoes a liver transplant.

113. A 50 year old woman who enjoys travelling to south East Asia presents with a four week history of lethargy and an annoying generalized purititis. She has now developed jaundice. Blood test reveal raised alkaline phosphatase and mild raised transaminases.

114. A 15 year old boy presents with jaundice and lethargy. His mother recalls that he had jaundice soon after birth and the only family history of note is his uncle who developed chest problems at a relatively early age.

115. A 60 year old "former hippy" male presents to the hepatology department for the results of tests to determine the cause of his cirrhosis. He is told that 30% of sufferers receive the same answer.

Women's health – Still births

116. Which of the following defines stillbirth?

    Select **ONE** option only.

    A. Babies born dead after 22 weeks
    B. Babies born dead after 24 weeks
    C. Babies born dead after 26 weeks
    D. Babies born dead after 28 weeks
    E. Babies born dead after 30 weeks

Respiratory problems – Peak expiratory flow rates

A. Ipratropium Bromide
B. Occupational asthma
C. Left ventricular failure
D. Salbutamol
E. Emphysema
F. Anaphylaxis
G. Asthma
H. Kyphosis
I. Normal
J. Beclomethasone
K. No medication

For each question below, select the **SINGLE MOST** appropriate answer from the options above. Each option can be used once, more than once or not at all.

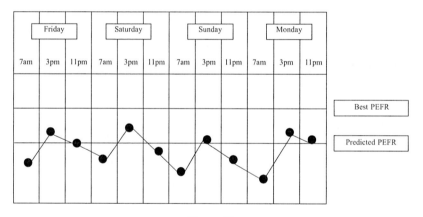

Figure 44

117. What does this peak flow chart demonstrate?
118. What, if anything, would you give to this patient initially?
119. If there was a significant difference between the peak expiratory flow rate (PEFR) on certain days what would this suggest?
120. If this patient became very breathless halfway through eating out at a restaurant what would be the most likely diagnosis?
121. If a patient's PEFR was consistently below 80% of predicted without diurnal variation what would be your diagnosis?

Men's health – Prostate cancer

122. In which group of people is prostate cancer more prevalent?

Select **ONE** option only.

A. Indian men
B. Chinese men
C. African men
D. European men
E. American men

Sexual health – Emergency pill

123. How effective is the emergency pill between 49-72 hours after unprotected sexual intercourse?

Select **ONE** option only.

A. 100%
B. 58%
C. 65%
D. 95%
E. 85%

Women's health – Malignancy

124. What is the most common malignancy in women?

Select **ONE** option only.

A. Breast cancer
B. Ovarian cancer
C. Cervical cancer
D. Lung cancer
E. Endometrial cancer

Management in primary care – Access to NHS care

125. A 40 year old refugee from Somalia has come to England. For how
long does he have to have been in the UK in order to be eligible
for NHS primary care?

Select **ONE** option only.

A. 2 months
B. 6 months
C. 3 months
D. 1 month
E. 4 months

Care of people with cancer and palliative care – Pain relief

126. A patient with lung cancer is being treated with 20mg morphine
sulphate bd. What dose of oral morphine should he be prescribed
for breakthrough pain?

Select **ONE** option only.

A. 6 mg
B. 8 mg
C. 5 mg
D. 7 mg
E. 4 mg

Research and academic activity – Statistics

127. In statistics what is the number needed to treat?

Select **ONE** option only.

A. 1 divided by the relative risk
B. 1 divided by the sensitivity
C. 1 divided by the absolute risk reduction
D. 1 divided by the specificity
E. 1 divided by the positive predictive value

ENT and facial problems – Epistaxis

128.   In epistaxis, what is the name of the group of vessels in the anterior septum which frequently bleed?

Select **ONE** option only.

A.   Broca's area
B.   Killian's area
C.   Cushing's area
D.   Little's area
E.   None of the above

Sexual health – Sexually transmitted infections

129.   Which if the following is most appropriate for treating uncomplicated Chlamydia?

Select **ONE** option only.

A.   Metronidazole 400 mg bd for 5 days
B.   Azithromycin 1 g stat
C.   Doxycycline 100 mg bd for 5 days
D.   Erythromycin 500 mg qds for 5 days
E.   None of the above

Metabolic problems – Goitres

A. Physiological goitre
B. Hashimoto's thyroiditis
C. Papillary adenocarcinoma
D. Folicular carcinoma
E. De Quervain's thyroiditis
F. Thyroid lymphoma
G. Grave's disease
H. Toxic goitre
I. Medullary carcinoma
J. Metastases
K. Thyroid cyst

For each case below, select the **SINGLE MOST** appropriate answer from the options above. Each option can be used once, more than once or not at all.

130. A patient presents with a tender goitre, fever and palpitations.
131. A 14 year old girl presents with a goitre but is otherwise asymptomatic.
132. A 20 year old woman presents with weight loss and palpitations for the previous 4 weeks. She has a smooth painless goitre.
133. A 50 year old who has a multinodular goitre has been losing weight recently and has lethargy.
134. A 48 year old woman has suffered from thyrotoxicosis for the last few months and a smooth goitre. She now has thickening of the skin over shins and low mood.

Care of people with mental health problems – Suicide

135. Which of the following is associated with the highest risk of suicide?

    Select **ONE** option only.

    A. Sertraline
    B. Citalopram
    C. Mirtazapine
    D. Paroxetine
    E. Venlafaxine

Sexual health – Contraception in menopause

136. A 51 year old woman is having symptoms of the menopause such as hot flushes and night sweats. She has come to see her GP to ask if she still needs to use contraception or not. What do you tell her?

Select **ONE** option only.

A. No contraception needed
B. Contraception needed until 12 months after last period
C. Contraception needed until 24 months after last period
D. Contraception needed for 6 months after her last period
E. None of the above

Cardiovascular problems – Chronic heart failure

A. Spironolactone
B. Beta blocker
C. ACE inhibitor
D. Digoxin
E. Angiotensin-II receptor antagonist
F. Furosemide

Below is an algorithm for the pharmacological management of symptomatic heart failure due to left ventricular dysfunction that has been adapted from NICE. Complete the numbered gaps with the **SINGLE MOST** appropriate option from the list above. Select **ONE** option only. Each option may be used, more than once or not at all.

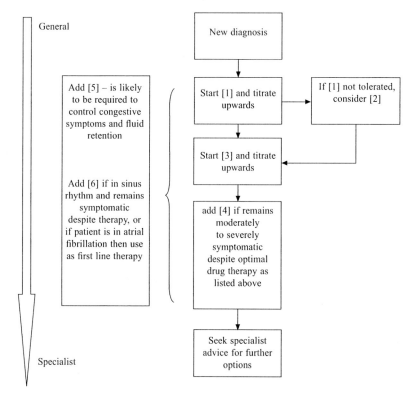

Figure 45

137. Blank 1
138. Blank 2
139. Blank 3
140. Blank 4
141. Blank 5
142. Blank 6

Personal and professional responsibilities – Cremation forms

143. Which of the following is true concerning Cremation 5?

Select **ONE** option only.

A. This should be completed by an independent doctor
B. This doctor should have been fully registered with the GMC for 2 years
C. There is no fee payable to the doctor
D. There is no need for the doctor to view the body
E. The doctor can be a relative of the deceased

Cardiovascular problems – Clinical trials

144. Patients with NYHA grade 4 who were already on an ACE inhibitor and loop diuretic were randomised to get either placebo or spironolactone in a trial. The results showed that the group with spironolactone added had a decreased all cause mortality rate. What trial does this refer to?

Select **ONE** option only.

A. ASCOT
B. 4S
C. HOT
D. RALES
E. UKPDS

Eye problems – Red Eye

A. Eye trauma
B. Herpes zoster infection
C. Acute closed-angle glaucoma
D. Bacterial conjunctivitis
E. Allergic conjunctivitis
F. Subconjunctival haemorrhage
G. Dry eye syndrome
H. Episcleritis
I. Scleritis
J. Contact lens use
K. Blepharitis

For each case below, select the **SINGLE MOST** appropriate diagnosis from the options above. Each option may be used once, more than once or not at all.

145. A 30 year old non-hypertensive, non-smoking man awakes one morning to find that that inner aspect of the white of his right eye has become red and bloodshot. There is no pain or visual loss and is otherwise well. He has had a cough for the last few days.

146. A 60 year old man with poorly controlled hypertension presents with a sudden onset, severely painful and red left eye associated with seeing haloes around lights and a left frontal headache. He also has nausea, vomiting and abdominal pain.

147. A 25 year old woman developed a red, right eye with no associated pain or visual problems. The superficial blood vessels were inflamed, but no conjunctival injection. The problem disappeared after 2 weeks whilst also taking ibuprofen.

148. An 8 year old boy has had red, sore, itchy eyes for the last 3 days. Mum says his eyelids are stuck together in the mornings and there is associated thick, yellow discharge. His temperature is 38.0 °C.

149. A 36 year old woman noticed some tingling around her left eye shortly followed by the onset of a blistering rash around the eye also affecting the tip of her nose. Her eye has now become red, painful and watery. Fluorescein staining revealed a central corneal ulcer with 'finger-like' projections.

Clinical governance

150. Which of the following is **NOT** part of clinical governance?

Select **ONE** option only.

A. Audit
B. Risk avoidance
C. Clinical effectiveness
D. Education/training
E. Confidentiality

Personal and professional responsibilities – Reporting deaths to coroner

151. Which of the following deaths does **NOT** need reporting to the coroner?

Select **ONE** option only.

A. Stillbirth
B. Sudden death
C. Industrial disease
D. Accidents
E. Expected death where doctor has seen patient within 10 days

Cardiovascular problems – Angina

A. Atenolol 100 mg od
B. Ramipril 1.25 mg od
C. Isosorbide mononitrate 20 mg bd
D. Glyceryl trinitrate (GTN) 400 micrograms sublingually prn
E. Emergency hospital admission
F. Nicorandil 5 mg od
G. Refer to a cardiology clinic
H. Amlodipine 5 mg od
I. Clopidogrel 75 mg od
J. Initiate warfarin therapy
K. Lacidipine 2 mg od

For each case below, select the **SINGLE MOST** appropriate next step in management from the options above. Each option may be used once, more than once or not at all.

152.   A 55 year old man, with known angina, gets 1 episode of chest pain per week lasting less than 2 minutes, on moderate exertion only. He already takes aspirin 75 mg od and atenolol100mg od.

153.   A 63 year old woman, with known left ventricular dysfunction is still getting angina pains despite taking a long-acting nitrate. She is not on any other medications.

154.   A 75 year old man, with known angina, is still getting symptoms despite use of atenolol, long-acting nitrate, a calcium-channel antagonist and nicorandil at maximum recommended doses.

155.   A 70 year old man sees you at the end of a busy Friday afternoon clinic. He had an episode of chest pain earlier this morning lasting for 4 hours. It radiates up his neck and to his jaw. He smokes 40 cigarettes per day. He is not on any regular medications. He is now pain free, his BP is 160/90 and cardio-respiratory exam is normal.

156.   An 80 year old woman with angina gets typical chest pains 3 to 4 times per week. She is already on atenolol and amlodipine at maximum doses. Her attacks occur on moderate exertion and are relieved by her sublingual GTN spray.

Healthy people: Promoting health and preventing disease – Smoking cessation

157. Concerning buproprion use, which of the following is **NOT** true?

Select **ONE** option only.

A. Contraindicated in those with history of seizures
B. Should be used in caution in those on anti-depressants
C. Max period of treatment is 7–9 weeks
D. Treatment starts 1–2 weeks before the target stop date
E. Can be used in those with eating disorders

Women's health – Postpartum mental health

158. Which of the following is **TRUE** about puerperal psychosis?

Select **ONE** option only.

A. It is associated with an inability to cope
B. It is screened for using the EPDS instrument
C. It occurs in about 10–15% of pregnancies
D. Symptoms last from a few hours to a few days
E. It is associated with paranoid delusions

Patient safety – Drug symbols

159. What does the following symbol in the BNF mean? ▼

Select **ONE** option only.

A. Controlled drug
B. Prescription-only medicine
C. Not prescribed on the NHS
D. Newly licensed medicine
E. A less suitable medicine to prescribe

Women's health – Alcohol in pregnancy

160. According to the NICE guideline March 2008 on Antenatal care which of the following is **FALSE?**

Select **ONE** option only.

  A. Advise women planning a pregnancy to avoid alcohol during the first 3 months
  B. If they choose to drink they should drink no more than one to two UK units of alcohol once or twice a week.
  C. Advise them to avoid getting drunk
  D. Binge drinking is allowed
  E. None of the above

Care of people with learning difficulties – Learning disability

  A. No learning disability
  B. Fragile X syndrome is likely cause
  C. Mild learning disability
  D. Down's syndrome is likely cause
  E. Moderate learning disability
  F. Foetal head injury during delivery is likely cause
  G. Severe learning disability
  H. Maternal recreational drug use in pregnancy is likely cause
  I Profound learning disability

For each intelligence quotient (IQ) score below, select the most appropriate statement from the list above. Select **ONE** option only.

161. IQ: 65
162. IQ: 105
163. IQ: 46
164. IQ: 15
165. IQ: 33

Rheumatology/Musculoskeletal system – Back pain

166. Which of the following is **NOT** a red flag sign of back pain?

Select **ONE** option only.

A. Loss of weight
B. History of cancer
C. Non-mechanical pain
D. Steroid use
E. Age 40

Men's health – Testicular problems

167. Which of the following requires immediate referral to hospital?

Select **ONE** option only.

A. Epididymo-orchitis
B. Epididymal cyst
C. Testicular torsion
D. Varicoele
E. Hydrocoele

Skin problems – Rashes

A. Lichen simplex
B. Lichen planus
C. Keratosis pilaris
D. Intertrigo
E. Tinea manuum
F. Bullous pemphigoid
G. Pemphigus
H. Hidradenitis suppurativa
I. Psoriasis
J. Kerion
K. Melasma

For each rash described, select the **SINGLE MOST** likely diagnosis. Each option may be used once, more than once or not at all.

168. A 23 year old flight attendant complains of itchy raised lesions around his elbow creases and on his palms and soles. He also has a white, lace-patterned rash inside his mouth.

169. A 28 year old woman has a three year history of recurrent nodules and abscesses in her axillae and groins.

170. A 92 year old nursing home resident has erupted in large, tense blisters on his limbs, trunk and flexures. There are also a few similar lesions in his mouth.

171. A 32 year old woman, with known myasthenia gravis, presents with fragile, superficial blisters on her scalp, face, back, chest and flexures.

172. A 15 year old Afro-Caribbean boy has a boggy, pustular swelling on the back of his scalp. He also has a temperature of 37.6 °C and a few tender, palpable cervical lymph nodes bilaterally.

Men's health – Testicular masses

173. Which of the following has a peak incidence in the age range 20–30 years old?

Select **ONE** option only.

A. Testicular teratoma
B. Testicular lymphoma
C. Testicular seminoma
D. Testicular cyst
E. None of the above

Women's health – Investigations for menorrhagia

174. According to the NICE guidelines on menorrhagia, what is the recommended first line investigation?

Select **ONE** option only.

A. Thyroid function tests
B. Haematinics
C. Full blood count
D. Oestrogen levels
E. None of the above

Metabolic problems – Osteoporosis

175. According to the NICE guidelines on secondary prevention of osteoporosis, who should **NOT** be on an oral bisphosphonate?

Select **ONE** option only.

A. 78 year old woman who has not had a DEXA scan
B. 67 year old woman with confirmed osteoporosis on her DEXA scan
C. A 58 year old woman with a T score of –2.6 and a BMI <20
D. A woman with rheumatoid arthritis and confirmed osteoporosis on her DEXA scan
E. A woman with a family history of maternal hip fracture at the age of 70 and confirmed osteoporosis on her DEXA scan

Digestive problems – Management of abdominal pain

A. Diverticulitis
B. Inflammatory bowel disease
C. Irritable bowel syndrome
D. Appendicitis
E. Pancreatitis
F. Urinary tract infection
G. Bladder outflow obstruction
H. Intestinal obstruction
I. Acute cholangitis
J. Alcoholic hepatitis
K. Adhesions

For each case described, select the **SINGLE MOST** appropriate diagnosis from the options below. Each option can be used once, more than once or not at all.

176. A 31 year old previously fit and well man presents with a two day history of fever, worsening lower abdominal pain, vomiting and loss of appetite. On examination he has generalised lower abdominal tenderness with rebound tenderness and guarding in the right liliac fossa.

177. A 54 year old woman presents with a six hour history of vomiting and severe right sided, upper abdominal pain which 'bores' through to her back. She has recently been getting worsening right sided, upper abdominal pain occurring about one hour after eating meals.

178. A 16 year old girl presents with a three day history of feeling 'hot and cold', lower abdominal pain, a burning pain when she urinates and increased frequency of passing urine. Urine dipstick is positive for nitrites, leucocytes and shows a trace of protein.

179. A 63 year old man presents with a three week history of right, upper abdominal pain, vomiting, jaundice and weight loss. He admits to drinking over a 100 units of alcohol per week for several years. On examination he has tender hepatomegaly.

180. A 27 year old woman presents with a 6 month history of abdominal cramps which are relieved on defecation and associated with alternating constipation/diarrhoea. There is some mucous in her stool, but no blood. The cramps are worse after eating and then she feels bloated.

Rheumatology/Musculoskeletal system – Ottawa rules

181.   Which is **NOT** part of the Ottawa ankle rules?

Select **ONE** option only.

A.   Pain over the posterior edge of the lateral malleolus
B.   Pain at the base of the 5th metatarsal
C.   Unable to weight bear immediately after injury and still
D.   Pain at the navicular bone
E.   Swelling and bruising

Neurological problems – Headache

A. Glaucoma
B. Transient ischaemic attack
C. Cluster headache
D. Migraine
E. Subarachnoid haemorrhage
F. Brain tumour
G. Temporal arteritis
H. Drug rebound headache
I. Sinusitis
J. Hydrocephalus
K. Tension-like headache

For each case described, select the **SINGLE MOST** appropriate diagnosis from the options above. Each option may be used once, more than once or not at all.

182. A 24 year old woman complains of a constant pressure over her head for three days. It gets worse as the day goes on and she drinks 10 cups of caffeinated tea per day. She has similar attacks once a month and is well between attacks. She also has irritable bowel syndrome.

183. A 30 year old man gets an intense burning pain around his left eye three-four times per day which lasts one hour and is often worse at night and on drinking alcohol. His left eye goes red and waters during attacks. Attacks last about 6 weeks and occur once every year.

184. A 64 year old woman complains of pain in her jaw when she eats for the last two days. She also says it hurts when she brushes her hair and that her shoulders are stiff and painful in the mornings.

185. A 27 year old woman complains of episodes of experiencing a strange smell shortly followed by a right sided headache (lasts about one hour) that is severe and makes her feel nauseous and intolerant of bright lights. She needs to lie down in a dark room to ease the pain and is well in between attacks. Her mother has history of headaches too.

186. A 50 year old, normotensive man complains of a sudden onset, severe posterior headache ("like someone's hit round the back of my head"). He had had a similar, much less severe headache two to three weeks before. He now complains of a stiff neck and some vomiting.

Care of people with mental health problems –
Eating disorders

187. Which of the following is the missing part of the questionnaire below?

Select **ONE** option only.

1. Do you make yourself sick because you feel uncomfortably full?

   Yes or No

2. X?

   Yes or No

3. Have you recently lost more than one stone in a 3 month period?

   Yes or No

4. Do you believe yourself to be fat when others say you are too thin?

   Yes or No

5. Would you say that food dominates your life?

   Yes or No

A. Do you ever think about cutting down on how much you eat?
B. Do you ever feel guilty about what you eat?
C. Do you ever feel angry about how much you eat?
D. Do you ever feel annoyed about your weight?
E. Do you ever worry you have lost control over how much you eat?

Care of people with mental health problems –
Obsessive compulsive disorder

188. According to step 2: recognition and assessment of obsessive compulsive disorder in the NICE guidelines, which of the following is **NOT** a symptom associated with higher risk of OCD?

Select **ONE** option only.

A. Anxiety
B. Depression
C. Schizophrenia
D. Eating disorder
E. Alcohol use

Digestive problems – Management of dyspepsia

A. Urgent referral for endoscopy
B. Routine referral for endoscopy
C. Trial of proton-pump inhibitor (PPI)
D. Trial of Gaviscon (or alike)
E. 1 week of triple therapy (2 antibiotics + full-dose PPI)
F. 2 weeks of triple therapy followed by 2 months of full-dose PPI
G. Full blood count
H. Low-dose PPI as required
I. Urease breath test
J. Trial of misoprostol
K. Trial of H$_2$-antagonist

For each case described, select the **SINGLE MOST** appropriate next step in management from the options above. Each option may be used once, more than once or not at all.

189. A 28 year old woman complains of epigastric pain which rises up her chest for the last four months, and is worse when she lies down at night.

190. A 70 year old man has had retrosternal chest pain (worse after eating) since his mid-forties. His recent *Helicobacter pylori* faecal antigen test came back positive. He has no red flag symptoms.

191. A 58 year old woman has had new onset dyspepsia for the last two months.

192. A 42 year old man recently had an endoscopy which confirmed an *H. pylori* positive duodenal ulcer. His gastroenterologist has written to you, as you are his GP, and requested you prescribe appropriate medications to treat his duodenal ulcer.

193. A 38 year old woman had an endoscopy for anaemia and dyspepsia, and was found to have an *H. pylori* positive gastric ulcer. She had a course of *H. pylori* triple therapy and repeat endoscopy eight weeks later showed she was *H. pylori* negative. What management should she now receive?

Care of children and young people – immunisation schedule

A. Meningococcus type C (Men C) vaccine
B. Malarial Vaccine (MV)
C. Bacille Calmette-Guerin (BCG) vaccine
D. Hepatitis B vaccine
E. Pneumococcal Vaccine (PCV)
F. Measles, Mumps and Rubella (MMR) Vaccine
G. Human Papilloma Virus (HPV) vaccine
H. Diphtheria, Tetanus, Acellular Pertusis vaccine/Inactivated Polio vaccine (DTaP/IPV/ or dTaP/IPV)
I. Tetanus, Diphtheria (Td)
J. Influenza vaccine
K. No vaccination necessary

For each numbered blank space in the diagram below choose the correct answer from the above options. Each option can be used once, more than once or not at all.

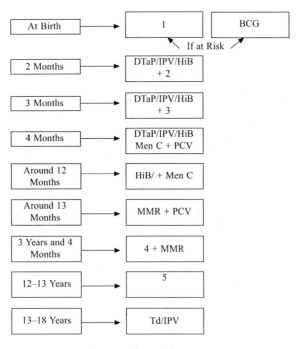

Figure 46

194. Blank 1
195. Blank 2
196. Blank 3
197. Blank 4
198. Blank 5

Rheumatology/Musculoskeletal system – Finger joint disorders

199. What type of deformity does the following picture show? Select **ONE** option only.

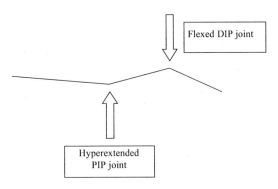

Figure 47

    A. Mallet finger
    B. Heberden's node
    C. Swan neck deformity
    D. Boutonniere deformity
    E. Bouchard's node

Care of children and young people – Paediatric drug calculations

200.   A Drug Y is given at a dose of 0.5 mg per kg three times a day. A boy weighs 20 kg.

Which of the following is the correct dose this boy should have? Select **ONE** option only.

A.   5 mg tds
B.   10 mg tds
C.   15 mg tds
D.   20 mg tds
E.   50 mg tds

Answer section: Mock Paper

1. B

   Side-effects of calcium-channel blockers commonly include: dizziness, headache, flushing and pitting oedema.

2. D

   NICE guidelines (2003) recommend that verapamil, diltiazem and short-acting dihydropridines such as nifedipine should be avoided. For more information see www.nice.org.uk

3. E

   Haemorrhagic strokes consist of approximately 20% of all strokes. There is usually no preceding transient ischaemic attack and hypertension is generally present. The clinical course is one that is rapidly progressive, signs of raised intra-cranial pressure are often present and the presence of blood will often show on CT brain scan. Ischaemic strokes tend to occur at night-time or when the patient is doing very little. There is usually a stepwise deterioration or the clinical course remains static.

4. D

   Alzheimer's disease is the commonest cause of dementia, followed by vascular and Lewy body dementia, which can all co-exist. NICE guidance on dementia (2006) states that neuroimaging should be used on all patients with suspected dementia. It recommends GP's should firstly do a dementia blood screen to exclude reversible causes (FBC, U&E, TFT, LFT, calcium, glucose, vitamin B_{12}, folate) and then patients are usually referred to a Memory Clinic. For more information see ww.nice.org.uk

5. C

   24 hours after a colonoscopy it is fine to fly

6. D

   For flights more than 2 hrs the restriction is increased from 24 hrs to 48 hrs

7. I

   5 days is the limit for this but the patient should be medically stable and an individual assessment is essential

8. J

   Pneumothorax is an absolute contraindication to air travel. Two weeks after successful drainage of the pneumothorax with full expansion of the lung should make it safe to fly.

9. B

   There is no restriction provided the haemoglobin is above 8.0 g/dL. If the haemoglobin is 7.5 g/dL or less then special assessment is needed

   See Civil Aviation Authority guidance on www.caa.co.uk/fitnesstofly for more information.

10. E

    Lower limb weakness or arthritis is a risk factor though.
    For more information see the NICE quick reference guide at http://www.nice.org.uk/nicemedia/pdf/CG021quickrefguide.pdf

11. B

    Here are some topical steroid creams categorised according to their degree of potency:

Mild steroid cream	Hydrocortisone 0.5–2.5%
Moderate steroid cream	Betamethasone valerate 0.025% (Betnovate RD) Clobetasone butyrate 0.05% (Eumovate)
Potent steroid cream	Betamethasone valerate 0.1% (Betnovate) Betamethasone diproprionate 0.025% (Propaderm)
Very potent steroid cream	Clobetasol proprionate 0.05% (Dermovate)

12. A

NICE urgent referral criteria for suspected colorectal cancer include:

- Aged ≥40 years old with rectal bleeding with a change of bowel habit towards looser stools and/or increased stool frequency persisting for ≥6 weeks.
- Aged ≥60 years old with rectal bleeding persisting for ≥6 weeks without change in bowel habit and without anal symptoms
- Aged ≥60 years old with change in bowel habit to looser stools and/or more frequent stools persisting for ≥6 weeks without rectal bleeding
- Any age with lower right abdominal mass with large bowel involvement
- Any age with a palpable rectal mass (not pelvic mass)
- Unexplained iron deficiency anaemia in men or non-menstruating women (Hb ≤11 g/dL in men and Hb ≤10 g/dL in non-menstruating women)

Diarrhoea is always more significant than constipation in terms of fast-tracking suspected lower GI cancer cases.

For more information see the NICE quick reference guide at http://www.nice.org.uk/nicemedia/pdf/CG027quickrefguide.pdf

13. B

3 main theories of learning:

(1) Cognitive theory – people learn by understanding, organising information, receiving feedback and by using learning aids (e.g. handouts).
(2) Behavioural theory – people learn by doing and repeating things in different situations and being rewarded for positive behaviour.
(3) Motivational theory – people learn naturally from their surroundings, they learn what they want to learn. They learn if they have some goal/purpose or if they are trying to out-compete someone.

14. C

The triptans are only used in acute attacks of migraines.

15. E

Xanthelasma are yellow flat plaques on the eyelids (most commonly the inner aspects) and can be associated with raised plasma lipid levels, familial hyperlipidaemia and corneal arcus. Management includes checking fasting lipid levels and cardiovascular risk assessment (may need a statin). Lesions can be left alone unless removal is wanted for cosmetic reasons – then cryocautery, applying trichloracetic acid or surgical excision can be tried.

16. C

This is due to compression of the radial nerve in the axilla or 'Saturday Night Palsy'.

17. G

When a portion of the thyroglossal duct remains patent it can form a cyst which is usually found between the isthmus of the thyroid gland and the hyoid cartilage, or just above the hyoid cartilage. They occur at any age with the majority between 15 and 30 years of age. They present usually as a painless, smooth, cystic, midline swelling in the region of the hyoid bone. They can become inflamed causing pain and swelling. On examination, the cyst rises as the patient swallows or protrudes their tongue.

18. H

A carotid aneurysm causes a pulsatile lateral neck swelling which does not move on swallowing. Treatment is with excision of the aneurysm.

19. D

A branchial cyst is an oval, mobile cystic mass that develops between the sternocleidomastoid and the pharynx, due to failure of the obliteration of the second branchial cleft in embryonic development. The cysts may enlarge following an upper respiratory tract infection. They are fluctuant but do not transilluminate and do not move on swallowing. They usually present in early adulthood. Treatment is with excision.

20. F

A pharyngeal pouch is a pulsion diverticulum of the pharyngeal mucosa through Killian's dehiscence, an area of weakness between the two parts of the inferior pharyngeal constrictor – the thyropharyngeus and the cricopharyngeus – at their posterior margin. It is usually not seen but if large enough it forms a midline swelling in the neck which gurgles on palpation. Other typical symptoms are dysphagia, aspiration, regurgitation and chronic cough.

21. B

Lymphoma is a neoplastic disorder of lymphoid tissue. There is Hodgkin's and Non-Hodgkin's lymphoma. In Hodgkin's there is contiguous spread between lymph nodes, whilst this is not present in Non-Hodgkin's. Reed-Sternberg cells are diagnostic of Hodgkin's. Hodgkin's has a better prognosis than Non-Hodgkin's. There is lymphadenopathy which is cervical or may be generalised. There may be alcohol related pain and the lymph nodes may be tender and feel rubbery. Night sweats and splenomegaly are also associated features.

22. A

This is distal tibial nerve entrapment or 'tarsal tunnel syndrome' (TTS) – the lower limb equivalent of carpal tunnel syndrome (CTS). Just as repeatedly tapping the median nerve reproduces CTS symptoms, tapping on the distal tibial nerve reproduces TTS symptoms.

23. E

Kayser-Fleischer rings are associated with Wilson's disease and are due to copper deposits where the cornea meets the sclera in Descemet's membrane.

24. A

Although the BMA gives copious advice on patient safety it is primarily the trade union for doctors and so is tasked with improving the working lives of their members. The GMC is paid for by doctors but has a duty to protect the public by maintaining competent standards of medicine. There are increasing numbers of lay members who sit on GMC panels which is a source of some controversy.

25. B

The Disability Discrimination Act 2005 requires GP partners to perform 'reasonable' actions to prevent discrimination against disabled doctors. There is no clear guidance as to what actions are deemed 'reasonable' but of all the answers providing disabled access seems the most reasonable. Answer A is an example of positive discrimination, answer C could be seen as harassment and even prejudice and answer D seems over generous considering counseling is free within the NHS.

26. E

Emphysema

27. D

Salbutamol

28. G

Asthma

29. C

Pneumothorax

30. B

Pulmonary Rehabilitation

31. C

There must be few false positives or negatives, there must be effective treatment at the stage of screening, the screening interval should be shorter than the time it takes for a disease to progress to an untreatable stage and the practice must always follow up the results of screening tests.

32. C

He is having a myocardial infarction secondary to cocaine ingestion. This is becoming more common with the rising use of cocaine as a recreational drug. This drug causes vasospasm in the coronary arteries and can lead to myocardial infarction and cardiac arrest.

33. F

You may be able to claim Bereavement Allowance if all of the following apply:

- you're a widow, widower or surviving civil partner aged 45 or over when your husband, wife or civil partner died
- you're not bringing up children
- you're under State Pension age (currently 60 for women and 65 for men)
- your late husband, wife or civil partner paid National Insurance contributions, or they died as a result of an industrial accident or disease

34. A

You can get disability living allowance if you have a physical or mental disability, or both, your disability is severe enough for you to need help caring for yourself or you have walking difficulties, or both, or you are under 65 when you claim

35. E

If you're working for an employer under a contract of service you are entitled to Statutory Sick Pay (SSP) if the following apply:

- you are sick for at least four days in a row (including weekends and bank holidays and days that you do not normally work)
- you're earning at least £95 a week

36. B

Attendance Allowance is for those that claim when they are above 65 years old

37. I

You can get Carer's Allowance if you're aged 16 or over and spend at least 35 hours a week caring for someone who gets either – Attendance Allowance, Disability Living Allowance (at the middle or highest rate for personal care) or Constant Attendance Allowance (at or above the normal maximum rate with an Industrial Injuries Disablement Benefit, or basic (full day) rate with a War Disablement Pension)

For more information on these benefits see www.direct.gov.uk

38. A

There is a good article in the British Journal of General Practice (Specialist skills for a generalist discipline: genetics in primary care. BJGP Feb 2009 vol. 59 No. 559). As GPs, we are the only truly generalist specialty in medicine which means we should have a good knowledge of most problems including genetics. We are not however required to prevent genetic disease (which is a controversial issue in itself) nor offer counselling.

39. C

Low dose Ramipril reduces microalbuminuria in people with type 1 diabetes without Hypertension (see *Diabetes Care* December 2000 vol. 23 no. 12 1823–1829). There is no reason to suspect pregnancy or UTI, as she is asymptomatic. A diuretic would be pointless.

40. B

This is otitis media. This is an inflammation of the middle ear, sometimes associated with an upper respiratory tract infection. Acute otitis media causes ear pain and tenderness, deafness and there may be a discharge from the ear. On otoscopy you may see a red, bulging ear drum. Management is with pain relief and symptoms should settle. Routine use of antibiotics is not recommended. The NICE guidelines on respiratory tract infections 2008 recommends the use of antibiotics for children younger than 2 with bilateral otitis media and children with otorrhoea who have acute otitis media.

A rare complication to look for is mastoiditis.

For more information see the NICE quick reference guide at http://www.nice.org.uk/nicemedia/pdf/CG69QRG.pdf

41. B

For more information see the NICE quick reference guide at http://www.nice.org.uk/nicemedia/pdf/CG012quickrefguide.pdf

42. C

The most common symptoms of lung cancer are shortness of breath, a persistent cough and weight loss. The most common cause of lung cancer is smoking and this man has at least a 32 year pack history (considering WW2 ended in 1945). As always remember; common things are common.

43. A

Section 2 allows for compulsory admission for assessment for 28 days. Application can be made by a relative or Approved Mental Health Professional (AMHP) and supported by 2 medical recommendations, one of which must be Section 12 approved.

44. E

5(4) allows detention of a patient by nursing staff for up to six hours while the doctor is found.

45. D

Section 5(2) allows for compulsory detention of someone already receiving inpatient treatment for up to a period of 72 hours by the doctor in charge of the case.

46. B

Section 3 is for treatment and lasts up to 6 months duration.

47. H

Section 136 allows the police to remove a person to a place of safety.

The acts allow detention of patients suffering with a mental disorder (any disorder or disability of the mind) in the interests of their own health and/or safety of others.

48. D

Pulmonary rehabilitation is recommended for patients whose symptoms are causing disability. You need to be aware of indications for long term oxygen use (i.e. pO_2 <7.3kPa unless other factors such as cor pulmonale). Read the British Thoracic Guidelines on oxygen therapy. Any patient with suicidal ideation should be investigated for psychiatric problems and offered help. Aiding suicide in any way is illegal and will result in you either getting a criminal record or being sent to prison.

49. B

Unfortunately this is rarely listened to but you should still give advice on healthy eating.

50. A

This is common in old age and more common in women. Risk factors are maternal hip fractures, osteoporosis, poor eye sight, unsteadiness and polypharmacy. A history of falls may be present. Signs on examination are external rotation of the hip, shortening of the leg and adduction of the leg. Urgent referral for an x-ray is needed.

51. A

Sensitivity is the true positives/(true positives plus false negatives)

52. B

Specificity is the true negatives/(true negatives plus false positives)

53. C

Positive predictive value is the true positives/(true positives plus false positives)

54. D

Negative predictive value is the true negatives/(true negatives plus false negatives)

The likelihood ratio for a positive test = sensitivity/ (1-specificity)

The likelihood ratio for a negative test = (1-sensitivity)/ specificity

55. C

The mode is the most frequent value

56. C

The median is the middle value

57. D

The mean is the sum of all the values divided by the number of values

58. F

The range is the difference between the lowest and highest values

59. C

Adhesive capsulitis (frozen shoulder) causes a painful, stiff shoulder with global restriction of movement, in particular external rotation. It typically occurs in those 40-60 years of age. There are three overlapping phases with it – freezing phase, adhesive phase and recovery phase. It may take two years from the onset of symptoms to full recovery. Management is with NSAIDs, physiotherapy and steroid injections. Sometimes referral to orthopaedics may be needed.

60. E

Gilbert's syndrome is an autosomal recessive disorder causing unconjugated hyperbilirubinaemia. It presents as jaundice shortly after birth, but then may go unnoticed for some years. Jaundice often occurs during inter-current illness. Increased fasting bilirubin confirms the diagnosis. No treatment is required. Crigler-Najjar syndrome is an inherited metabolic disorder presenting with neonatal jaundice where many patients die within first year of life from kernicterus (hyperbilirubinaemia causing brain damage). They often need phototherapy and/or phenobarbitone.

61. E

Practice-based commissioning (PBC) is about empowering GPs and other clinicians such as nurses, pharmacists and allied health professionals to shape the health and healthcare of local populations. 'Children' is not one of the components of the PBC budget formula. You need to be familiar with this concept. For more information on PBC go to www.dh.gov.uk

62. D

The odds ratio is the odds in the treatment group compared with the odds in the placebo group. In this case:

Odds of improved symptoms with drug B = 70/30 = 2.3333

Odds of improved symptoms with placebo = 20/60 = 0.3333

Therefore the odds ratio is 2.3333/0.3333 = 7

63. E

This is not routinely required unless there are risk factors or points in the clinical history indicate need. The same applies to HIV. Routine examination of cerebrospinal fluid is also not required. For more information see the NICE quick reference guide at http://www.nice.org.uk/nicemedia/pdf/CG042quickrefguide.pdf

64. E

If there is a clear history of mechanical locking then referral for arthroscopic lavage and debridement should be done. No other symptom warrants referral. For more information see the NICE quick reference guide at http://www.nice.org.uk/nicemedia/pdf/ CG59quickrefguide.pdf

65. C

A simple faint does not require you to stop driving. If a patient has had a MI then they need to stop driving for 4 weeks, if they have had an angioplasty then for 1 week, an epileptic needs to be seizure free for 12 months before they can drive and if a pacemaker is inserted then they should stop driving for a week. For more information see the DVLA website at www.dvla.gov.uk

66. C

Urinary incontinence is the inappropriate and involuntary loss of urine which can be objectively demonstrated. Stress incontinence is the involuntary loss of urine on effort, exertion, sneezing or coughing. Urge incontinence is the involuntary loss of urine accompanied or immediately preceded by urgency. Mixed incontinence is the involuntary loss of urine associated with both urgency and exertion, effort, sneezing or coughing. NICE recommends a trial of supervised pelvic muscle floor training of at least three months duration as first line treatment of stress or mixed incontinence. For women with urge or mixed incontinence bladder training for at least six weeks should be offered as first line treatment. For more information see the NICE quick reference guide at http://www. nice.org.uk/nicemedia/pdf/word/CG40quickrefguide1006.pdf

67. E

Implanon is a long acting reversible contraceptive. It is licensed for 3 years and it requires a trained professional to both insert and remove it. It works by preventing ovulation. A third of women stop using it because of irregular bleeding. Fifty percent of women have either frequent, infrequent or prolonged bleeding with it. For more information see the NICE quick reference guide at http://www. nice.org.uk/nicemedia/pdf/cg030quickrefguide.pdf

68. **A**

Cerazette (desogestrel) is a progesterone only pill. These should be taken everyday at the same time. Cerazette works by inhibiting ovulation. Unlike the traditional progesterone only pills it has a 12 hour window for missed pills and not three hours. If a woman vomits within two hours of taking a pill she should take another one as soon as possible. The efficacy of progesterone only pills is not reduced by non-liver enzyme-inducing antibiotics and so additional contraceptive protection is not needed.

For more information see the Faculty of Sexual and Reproductive Healthcare site at www.ffprhc.org.uk/admin/uploads/CEUGuidanceProgestogenOnlyPill08.pdf

69. **F**

This is bacterial vaginosis so needs treating with metronidazole

70. **A**

An inadequate sample needs repeating immediately

71. **B**

Mild dyskaryosis is consistent with CIN 1 and needs a repeat smear in 6 months.

72. **E**

Moderate and severe dyskaryosis (consistent with CIN II and CIN III respectively) require referral for colposcopy.

73. **D**

Within the cervical screening programme women between the ages of 25–49 have smear tests every 3 years and then every 5 years between the ages of 50–64.

For more information see the NHS cervical screening programme website at: www.cancerscreening.nhs.uk/cervical/

74. **D**

For sperm analysis 3 days of abstinence is needed before it. Normal values include:

- Volume ≥ 2 ml
- Motility ≥50%
- Morphology ≥15% normal forms
- Sperm concentration ≥20 million spermatozoa per ml
  For more information see www.gpnotebook.co.uk

75. A

The NICE guidelines on referral for suspected cancer say that if the man is 50 or above with a unilateral, firm subareolar mass with or without nipple distortion or associated skin changes should be referred urgently.

For more information see the NICE quick reference guide at http:// www.nice.org.uk/nicemedia/pdf/CG027quickrefguide.pdf

76. E

Male sterilisation, vasectomy is a simple procedure in which part or all of the vas deferens is excised, which is done under local anaesthetic as an outpatient. The failure rate is 1 in 2000. Two negative specimens 3 months after the procedure one month apart are needed in order to say the patient is sterile. Wound haematoma and infection can occur and chronic testicular pain can be a late complication.

For more information see www.gpnotebook.co.uk

77. C

This is the correct starting dose of methotrexate. See BNF for more information.

78. D

Post traumatic stress disorder is a reaction to a stressful event (war, rape, natural disaster) in which there is a delayed onset of symptoms and intense and prolonged psychological disturbance. The prevalence in the population is about 2–3%. Symptoms typically include: hyperarousal, hypervigilance, sleep problems, poor concentration, avoidance (avoiding people, places or situations associated with the event) and re-experiencing the event in flashbacks, nightmares and intrusive imagery. Obsessions are not a feature. If symptoms are mild and have been present for less than four weeks after the trauma, watchful waiting is an approach. For severe PTSD trauma-focused cognitive behavioural therapy should be offered. Drug treatments should not be used as first line treatment but may be used in adults that do not want to engage in trauma-focused CBT. If this is the case then paroxetine or mirtazipine are used.

For more information see the NICE quick reference guide at http:// www.nice.org.uk/nicemedia/pdf/CG026quickrefguide.pdf

79. H

In de Quervain's disease, the sheath containing extensor pollicis brevis and abductor pollicis longus tendons becomes thickened and inflamed. It is more common in women and in 30–50 year olds. Gardening is often associated with this pain on the radial side of the wrist. There is pain on forced adduction and flexion of the thumb and over the radial styloid. Finkelstein's test where with the thumb flexed across the palm of the hand you ask the patient to move the wrist into flexion and ulnar deviation reproduces the pain of de Quervain's tenosynovitis. Management is with a thumb splint, steroid injection or surgery if needed.

80. B

Medial epicondylitis (Golfer's elbow) is caused by inflammation of the flexor origin at the medial humeral epicondyle, where there is pain and tenderness. It is less common than Tennis elbow. There is medial elbow pain on resisted wrist pronation. Rest, NSAIDs and avoidance of activity that precipitates pain is advised. Steroid injections may help settle cases and physiotherapy and an elbow brace may also help.

81. A

Lateral epicondylitis (Tennis elbow) is caused by inflammation of the common extensor origin, at the lateral epicondyle of the humerus. It is a common cause of elbow pain. Tennis is one cause but there others. Pain is localised to the front of the lateral epicondyle. Movements such as shaking hands or lifting the wrist with the forearm pronated worsen the pain. Resisted wrist extension causes lateral elbow pain. Rest, NSAIDs and avoidance of activities that worsen symptoms is advised. Steroid injections and surgery may be needed. Physiotherapy is the best long term treatment option.

82. C

Carpal tunnel is compression of the median nerve as it passes under the flexor retinaculum. Patients get painful paraesthesiae of the fingers and hands, thenar muscle wasting and pain in the radial 3½ digits of the hand. Females are affected 3 times more than men. The majority of patients are between 40–60 years old. Symptoms are worse at night and relief can be had from shaking the hands or hanging them over the bed. There is a positive Phalen's test where forced wrist flexion causes exacerbation of symptoms. Tinel's test is positive where tapping of the carpal tunnel causes paraesthesiae. Nerve conduction tests show a reduced conduction velocity. Management includes night splints, steroid injections and surgery to divide the flexor retinaculum.

83. E

A ganglion is a cyst arising from a joint or tendon sheath, occurring most commonly around the wrist. It presents in a young adult with a smooth, firm, painless lump, usually on the back of the wrist. It may disappear on its own without any treatment. If the lump is troublesome then it may be aspirated and can be injected with steroids.

84. A

Anti-rhesus (anti-D) immunoglobulin should be given after delivery to all Rh-negative women where the baby's blood group cannot be determined and following the birth of a Rh-positive infant, immediately or within 72 hours. Anti-D prophylaxis is offered to all non-sensitised pregnant women who are RhD negative given as two doses at 28 and 34 weeks gestation. Anti-D should be given to all non-sensitised RhD negative women who have a threatened miscarriage after 12 weeks or an incomplete or complete miscarriage after 12 weeks gestation, all non-sensitised women with an ectopic pregnancy, all non-sensitised women having a therapeutic termination regardless of gestational age and after sensitizing events like amniocentesis, chorionic villous sampling, external cephalic version, antepartum haemorrhage.

For more information see the NICE quick reference guide at http://www.nice.org.uk/nicemedia/pdf/CG062QuickRefGuide.pdf, the RCOG guidance on Greentop 22 at: www.rcog.org.uk/womens-health/clinical-guidance/use-anti-d-immunoglobulin-rh-prophylaxis-green-top-22 and also: www.gpnotebook.co.uk

85. E

The combined pill contains both oestrogen and progesterone. It works by inhibiting ovulation. It is effective immediately if started on day 1 of the period up to day 5, otherwise additional contraception is required for 7 days. It can be used after 21 days postpartum. Women should be counselled about how it works, how to take it, missed pills rules, side effects and interactions.

Absolute contraindications include:

- Aged ≥35 and smoking ≥15/day
- BMI ≥40
- <6 weeks postpartum
- Current VTE (on anticoagulant) or past history
- Cardiovascular disease
- Uncontrolled hypertension
- Known thrombogenic mutations
- Major surgery
- Stroke
- Migraine with aura
- Current breast cancer
- Active viral hepatitis
- Diabetes

For more information see the Faculty of Sexual and Reproductive Healthcare website at www.ffprhc.org.uk/admin/uploads/FirstPrescCombOralContJan06.pdf

See the UK Medical Eligibility Criteria (UKMEC) criteria for more information on the contraindications at www.ffprhc.org.uk/admin/uploads/298_UKMEC_200506.pdf

86. B

The GMS contract is made between the practice and the local PCT. It is a nationally agreed, locally managed contract. The services provided by the practice are divided into essential services, additional services and enhanced services. Essential services include the day-to-day medical care of the practice population, general management of patients who are terminally ill and chronic disease management. Additional services include cervical screening, vaccinations and immunisations, contraceptive services, child health surveillance, maternity services and certain minor surgical procedures.

87 C

This is the only correct option from the list. Prevalence is a measure of the proportion of people that have a disease at one point in time or over some period of time. Incidence is the number of new cases of a disease within the population over a specific time period. Interpretation of data from charts like this is a nice way to get a mark.

88. A

The GMC is going to be in charge of the new revalidation that is going to start later this year. There will be three choices, you can either be registered with a licence to practise (£410), or you can be registered without a licence to practise (£145) or you can no longer be registered. For more information go to www.gmc-uk.org

89. D

Infertility is the failure of conception after 12 months in a couple having regular, unprotected normal intercourse at least twice a week. The age is 35 and above that will need investigation for primary infertility.

90. D

The Kings Fund is an independent charitable organisation that works to improve healthcare in the UK through research and health policy analysis amongst other activities.

91. B

The green book is a department of health document that details the available range of immunizations against infectious diseases.

92. G

This is secondary prevention as he already had diabetes and now you are attempting to prevent the complications of this by making sure that he is monitored annually. There are NICE guidelines on this and the management of patients with diabetes is part of the quality outcome framework.

93. I

The Wilson-Junger Criteria states that the disease being screened for should have effective treatment available and management in the early stages should affect prognosis.

94. F

This patient's health beliefs mean that he goes against medical advice. Your job is to persuade (not coerce) the patient of the need for safe sex procedures.

95. B

This is the most suitable choice in pregnancy. See the BNF for list of medications that should not be used in pregnancy.

96. A

A type 1 error is when you reject the null hypothesis when it is true. A type 2 error is when you accept the null hypothesis when it is false. The power of a study is the probability of correctly rejecting the null hypothesis when it is false. Therefore the power of a study is 1- probability of a type 2 error.

97. C

This is not one of the four main principles. Autonomy is about our own self rule and ability to make our own decisions. Beneficence means to do good and non-maleficence means do no harm. Justice means to do what is fair.

98. B

This is the description of calculating the mean. You need to add all the values up and divide by the total number of values.

99. G

The HPV vaccine is very controversial as some people believe it will promote promiscuity amongst young people. There is also some controversy as to which vaccine was chosen for distribution on the NHS. Cervarix is offered by the NHS and protects against HPV 16/18 (providing some protection against cervical cancer) whereas Gardasil protects against HPV 6/11/16/18 and so provides protection against cervical cancer and genital warts.

100. J

The Influenza vaccine is indicated for young people who are at risk of catching the infection, those over 65 years of age and for those living or working in places in which there is a greater risk than normal of catching the virus e.g. healthcare workers

101. F

In 1998, a paper published in the Lancet suggested a link between Autism and the triple MMR vaccination. This paper was later discredited and 10 of the 12 co-authors retracted their claims. Following this the MMR uptake has dropped and there has been an increase in measles outbreaks.

102. K

Unfortunately a malarial vaccine does not exist at present but would potentially save millions of lives. Anti-malarial prophylaxis, mosquito nets and safe practice are the only methods of protection at present.

103. I

This child has only had his first three tetanus vaccinations and will require a booster. If a child had been fully immunized and has received his five doses of tetanus vaccine they usually will not need another booster unless 10 years later they decide to travel to a remote location where they could potentially get a very dirty wound and not receive anti-serum. Otherwise human tetanus immunoglobulin can be given (whether immunised or not) in cases where there is a high chance of tetanus contamination in a wound.

104. C

When the relative risk is greater than one this means the intervention increases the risk of the outcome being studied. If it is less than one it decreases the risk. If it is 0 there is no relationship.

105. D

Osteoporosis is defined as a bone mineral density > 2.5 SDs below the mean. In contrast to osteomalacia there is still normal bone mineralization. It increases with age and is more common in women (3:1). By the third decade there is a gradual loss of bone mass. By the age of 70 one third of Caucasian women will have had at least one vertebral fracture. About one fifth of women will have had a hip fracture by the age of 90. Investigation is with DEXA scan if <75 and to exclude other causes. Management:

- If ≥75 treat without a DEXA scan once all non-osteoporotic causes of fracture have been ruled out
- If 65–74 treat if DEXA scan confirms osteoporosis
- If <65 and a very low BMD (T score ≤–3) or T score ≤–2.5 and one of the following – low BMI (<19) or height loss >3 cm, FH of maternal hip fracture aged <75, untreated premature menopause, medical conditions associated with bone loss such as Rheumatoid arthritis, Ankylosing Spondylitis, Type 1 Diabetes.

Bisphosphonates are the mainstay of treatment and prevention.

For more information see www.gpnotebook.co.uk

106. C

The number needed to treat is calculated by dividing 1 by the absolute risk reduction. The absolute risk reduction is 20/100 – 5/100 which = 0.15. 1/0.15 is rounded up to 7.

107. A

The others do not justify removal from the practice. Violence (physical or verbal abuse) towards doctors, staff, premises or patients, and crime and deception are also reasons that justify removal from the practice list.

108. C

SCOFF is a questionnaire designed to screen for anorexia or bulimia. There are 5 questions requiring a 'yes' or 'no' answer, with one point for every 'yes' answer. If there is a score of ≥2 it indicates a likely case of anorexia or bulimia. The other options are all alcohol questionnaires.

109. D

This is an enzyme inhibitor. The others are all inducers. Other enzyme inhibitors include: cimetidine, isoniazid, sulphonamides, ketoconazole, sodium valproate, allopurinol.

110. E

This is the lowest level of evidence. Here is a table of the evidence levels:

Grade	Evidence level	Where evidence from
A	Ia Ib	Meta analysis of randomised controlled trials At least one randomised controlled trial
B	IIa IIb III	At least one well designed controlled study without randomisation e.g case controlled study, cohort study At least one other type of well designed quasi experimental study Well designed non experimental descriptive studies such as comparative studies, correlation studies and case studies
C	IV	Expert committee reports or opinions and/or clinical experience of respected authorities

111. D

Haemochromotosis causes iron deposits in the heart, liver, joints, pituitary gland and pancreas. It is diagnosed by raised transferring saturation levels and sometimes by tissue biopsy. It is either primary due to the HFE gene or secondary due to iron overload caused by various blood disorders or excessive iron intake.

112. C

This causes copper deposition in the cornea (Kayser-Fleischer rings), liver, brain and kidneys.

113. G

Inherited through maternal mitochondrial DNA this causes an obstructive pattern of liver failure.

114. F

This autosomal recessive disorder also causes early onset emphysema.

115. A

In 30% of sufferers of cirrhosis a cause is not found.

116. B
Stillbirth is a foetus delivered after 24 weeks gestation with no signs of life after complete expulsion.

117. G

118. D

119. B

120. F

121. E

122. C
Prostate cancer is the second most common cancer in men in the UK. It is the second most common cause of death of cancer in men. The most common age of presentation is between 65–85 years of age and it is rare before 50 years. The majority are well differentiated adenocarcinomas. Family history is a risk factor and so is being Afro-Carribean. Patients may be asymptomatic or they may have symptoms such as bladder outlet obstruction, haematuria or haematospermia, pain and constipation. There may be features of metastatic disease also. Rectal examination may reveal a stony hard, irregular prostate with obliteration of the median sulcus. Investigations include PSA and a transrectal ultrasound of prostate with needle biopsy. Treatment depends on the extent of disease and includes watchful waiting, radiotherapy, hormone treatment and surgery.

123. B
Levonorgestrel should be given as a 1.5 mg single dose as soon as possible after unprotected sexual intercourse within 72 hours. After 72 hours the efficacy is reduced and it can be considered but it is not licensed for this. Within 24hrs it is 95% effective, within 48hrs 85% and within 72hrs 58%. If the patient vomits within 2 hours of taking the pill they need to have a repeat dose. If the next period is lighter or heavier than usual or; is more than 7 days late or; if they have abdominal pain they should be advised to take a pregnancy test and return for advice.

For more information see the Faculty of Sexual and Repro-ductive Healthcare website at www.ffprhc.org.uk/admin/uploads/449_ EmergencyContraceptionCEUguidance.pdf

124. A

   Breast cancer is the most common malignancy in women

125. B

   People are entitled to primary care if they are a resident, meaning that they will be in the UK for at least 6 months. It is not based upon nationality or national insurance contributions.

126. D

   The breakthrough dose of morphine should be 1/6 the total daily dose of morphine. To convert morphine to oxycodone you need to divide by 2. To convert morphine to diamorphine you need to divide by 3.
   For more information see the SIGN guidelines at http://www.sign.ac.uk/guidelines/fulltext/106/index.html

127. C

   The number needed to treat is 1/the absolute risk reduction

128. D

   Epistaxis is common and has a bimodal age distribution common in children less than 10 and also in adults above 50. It is more common in men. In the young the blood comes from Little's area which is a highly vascular area at the anterior border of the nasal septum. With age the site of bleeding becomes more posterior. Risk factors include irritants such as cigarette smoke, colds and allergies, deviated nasal septum, medical conditions such as hypertension and haemophilia, drugs and alcohol. Management depends on severity and can include nasal cautery, packing and surgery.

129. B

   Chalmydia is treated with either doxycycline 100 mg twice a day for 7 days or azithromycin 1 g stat. If the above is contraindicated then you can use erythromycin 500 mg twice a day for 10–14 days or ofloxacin 200 mg twice a day for 14 days or 400 mg once a day for 7 days. See www.bashh.org/guidelines for more information.

130. E

   De Quervain's thyroiditis is thought to be viral in origin. It is treated by NSAIDs and sometimes requires corticosteroids.

131. A

   Physiological goiters occur most commonly in women aged 15 – 25 years old. They are smooth and painless and usually resolve.

132. G

Grave's disease is caused by thyroid stimulating IgG immunoglobulins. It causes hyperthyroidism, pretibial myxoedema and also directly attacks the orbital tissues causing oedema, proptosis, opthalmoplegia. It is a relapsing and remitting disease.

133. D

Folicular carcinoma. The most common (90%) forms of thyroid cancer are called differentiated thyroid cancers which are divided in to papillary (80%) and follicular adenocarcinoma (10%). Five percent of patients have medullary thyroid cancer which can be familial. In the elderly two rare types occur; thyroid lymphoma and anaplastic thyroid cancer.

134. B

Hashimoto's thyroiditis is the most common cause of hypothyroidism in non-iodine deficient areas. It is an autoimmune disorder characterized by the infiltration of lymphocytes and plasma cells in the thyroid.

135. A

Sertraline is the medication with the highest risk of suicide. Risk factors for suicide are being male, increasing age, divorced > widowed > never married > married, social isolation, history of deliberate self-harm, depression, alcohol or substance misuse, personality disorder, schizophrenia, serious medical illness, recent admission or discharge to psychiatric hospital, jobs (doctors).

136. B

If over 50 then contraception is needed for 12 months, if under 50 years old then it is needed for 2 years

137. Blank 1 – C

138. Blank 2 – E

139. Blank 3 – B

140. Blank 4 – A

141. Blank 5 – F

142. Blank 6 – D

For more information see the NICE quick reference guide at: http://guidance.nice.org.uk/CG5/Guidance/pdf/English

143. A

Cremation 5 (formerly cremation C) must be completed by an independent doctor to the one who completed cremation 4 and must not be connected to the patient in any way. They should have been fully registered with the GMC for 5 years. There is a fee payable for completing this form. See the new guidance at www.justice. gov.uk/guidance/cremation.htm for more information.

144. D

This describes the RALES study. Be familiar with the major studies and trials as they can come up in some form as a question.

145. F

Subconjunctival haemorrhage – painless and reddening of the eye under the conjunctiva. It can be due to minor trauma or coughing/ sneezing. No treatment required as subsides by itself (but check blood pressure isn't high). Often noticed on waking in the morning, it is more concerning if bilateral and/or recurrent.

146. C

Acute closed-angle glaucoma – raised intraocular pressure due to blockage of aqueous outflow. Condition may present as sudden visual loss with painful, red eye, seeing haloes around lights and a frontal headache. Miosis (pupil constriction) will abort the attack i.e. if patient goes into dark room or closes their eyes. The eye is stony hard, with a semi-reactive, dilated pupil and hazy cornea. Refer urgently to on-call ophthalmologist and treatment is with topical pilocarpine and surgical or laser iridectomy to improve aqueous outflow.

147. H

Episcleritis – mildly painful, inflammation of the superficial blood vessels in the thin layer which overlies the sclera (episclera). Usually self-limiting and relieved with NSAIDs. Scleritis is generally more painful than episcleritis.

148. D

Bacterial conjunctivitis – purulent discharge and eyelashes are stuck together in the morning. Eyes are itchy and gritty rather than painful. Treatment is with topical antibiotic drops or ointment (e.g. chloramphenicol or fusidic acid)

149. B
Herpes zoster – may get numbness or tingling around the eye followed by eruption of a blistering rash. If the tip of the nose is affected, then this signifies involvement of nasociliary branch of trigeminal nerve, and so the eye is much more likely to be affected. The eye can be painful, red and watery. Refer urgently to on-call ophthalmologist. Need to exclude a dendritic ulcer and start oral antiviral therapy.

150. E
Clinical governance is a framework through which NHS organisations are accountable for continuously improving the quality of their services and safeguarding high standards of care by creating an environment in which excellence in clinical care will flourish. Confidentiality is not part of clinical governance.

151. E
Deaths where the doctor has not seen the patient in 14 days need reporting to the coroner. Other deaths that should be reported to the coroner include:

- Unexpected or sudden deaths
- Deaths arising from ill treatment
- Unknown cause of death
- Suicide
- Accidents and injuries
- Industrial injury or disease
- If a death occurs within 24 hrs of hospital admission
- Stillbirths
- Poisoning
- Death occurred during an operation or before recovery from the effect of an anaesthetic

152. D

153. H

154. G

155. E

156. C

GTN spray 'as required' is suitable if angina attacks are mild and infrequent (<2 attacks per week). These further medications should be added stepwise starting with (a) atenolol (b) long-acting dihydropyridine calcium-channel blocker (e.g. amlodipine) and (c) long-acting nitrate.

157. E

Buproprion is a norepinephrine and dopamine reuptake inhibitor and nicotinic antagonist. It should be started 1–2 weeks before the patient target stop date. There is a small risk of seizures with it. It is contraindicated in epilepsy, pregnancy, breast feeding and is relatively contraindicated in those with an eating disorder.

For more information see the NICE quick reference guide at http://www.nice.org.uk/nicemedia/pdf/PH010quickrefguide1.pdf

158. E

Puerperal psychosis is a rare complication of pregnancy with an incidence of 1–2/1000. It is associated with delusions, hallucinations, a clouding of consciousness and the onset is usually 3–4 days postpartum. Make sure you know the difference between this and postpartum blues and postnatal depression.

159. D

This symbol means a newly licensed medicine. See the BNF for information about the other common symbols used.

160. D

Binge drinking is not advised. The others are all true. For more information see the NICE quick reference guide at http://www.nice.org.uk/nicemedia/pdf/CG062QuickRefGuide.pdf

161. C

162. A

163. E

164. I

165. **G**

Intelligence quotient scores are one way of classifying learning disability:

> 70	No learning disability
50–69	Mild learning disability
35–49	Moderate learning disability
20–34	Severe learning disability
< 20	Profound learning disability

166. **E**

Red flag signs are age <20 and >55, non-mechanical back pain, HIV, taking steroids, unwell, weight loss, widespread neurology, past history of carcinoma, thoracic pain, structural deformity.

167. **C**

Testicular torsion is an emergency and needs immediate referral to hospital in case surgery is needed.

168. **B**

Lichen planus – itchy, shiny, mauve, flat-topped papules of unknown cause which sometimes have white streaks on the surface (Wickham's striae) and can affect the mucous membranes.

169. **H**

Hidradenitis suppurativa – disease affecting the sweat glands in the axillae, groins and perineum characterised by painful nodules, papules and abscesses. Treatment is usually with long courses of antibiotics (like in acne) or with surgical excision.

170. **F**

Bullous pemphigoid – acquired autoimmune condition which is characterised by presence of large, tense blisters (commonest cause of blistering rash in elderly). IgG antibodies to basement membrane found in blood. Blisters occur at dermal-epidermal junction.

171. **G**

Pemphigus – autoimmune disease characterised by fragile blisters within the epidermis of skin and mucous membranes. This affects a lot more younger people than bullous pemphigoid. IgG antibodies target cell surface antigens on keratinocytes.

172. J
Kerion – boggy, inflammatory swelling with pustules which occurs on the scalp. Due to inflammatory reaction to dermatophyte infection, sometimes with super-added bacterial infection.

173. A
Testicular seminomas are more common between ages 30-40. Teratomas are more common between 20–30 years old. Lymphoma is more common in those aged 60–70 years old.

174. C
Investigations which are not recommended are serum ferritin, thyroid testing, direct and indirect menstrual blood loss measurements. For more information see the NICE quick reference guide at: http://www.nice.org.uk/nicemedia/pdf/CG44quickrefguide.pdf

175. C
The BMI needs to be less than 19

176. D
Appendicitis – usually occurs due to obstruction of the appendix (e.g. due to faecolith). Characterised by central abdominal discomfort which then spreads to right iliac fossa and becomes severe and constant. There may be peritonism. Associated with nausea/vomiting, loss of appetite, occasionally diarrhoea and patients often wish to lie still.

177. E
Pancreatitis – characterised by upper abdominal pain (often radiates through to the back), nausea and vomiting. Alcohol in men and gallstones in women are the commonest causes. Abdominal wall discolouration (Grey-Turner's and Cullen's signs) is virtually pathognomonic.

178. F
Urinary tract infection (UTI) – may present with fever, dysuria and urgency. For uncomplicated UTI in women, treat with oral antibiotics for 5 days.

179. J
Alcoholic hepatitis – may present with fatigue, weight loss, anorexia, fever and tender hepatomegaly. Other signs of chronic liver disease or liver failure may also be present (e.g. spider naevi, ascites, encephalopathy, liver flap, etc.)

180. C

Irritable bowel syndrome (IBS) – chronic, relapsing condition characterised by alternating bowel habit and abdominal pain or discomfort which may be relieved by defecation. Mucous in stool may also occur (no blood). IBS is a diagnosis of exclusion as symptoms may overlap with inflammatory bowel disease and Coeliac disease. Treat with isphaghula husk (if constipation-predominant IBS), loperamide (if diarrhoea-predominant) or peppermint oil.

181. E

People should be referred for an ankle x-ray if there is pain in the malleolar area and,

- Bone tenderness at the posterior tip of the lateral malleolus or;
- Bone tenderness at the posterior tip of the medial malleolus or;
- Patient is unable to weight bear at the time of the injury and when seen.

182. K

Tension-like headache – often described as a bilateral, mild to moderate intensity, pressure feeling or 'tight band' around head. Sometimes felt in frontal or occipital areas. Symptoms may get worse throughout the day. There is no aura or neurological deficit and patients are generally well in themselves otherwise.

183. C

Cluster headache – severe pain around one eye which can last up to 2 hours with watering of the eye and nasal congestion. More common in middle-aged males and can be triggered by alcohol. Attacks can occur daily for 6–8 weeks and bouts occur every few months or years. Treatment is with oxygen, ergotamine (injectable or nasal form and nasal triptan sprays.

184. G

Temporal arteritis – vasculitis in elderly affecting medium-large sized arteries which may cause sudden loss of vision. Can get temporal artery tenderness, reduced temporal artery pulse or jaw claudication. Associated with polymyalgia rheumatica. ESR is high and if diagnosis is suspected, treat with high dose oral steroids (prednisolone 60–80 mg/day) until ESR result if available. But if visual loss is present, refer as emergency to on-call ophthalmologist.

185. D

Migraine – episodic headaches with no interval symptoms. Headaches are severe, pulsating and usually unilateral. There may be an aura or associated nausea, vomiting, photophobia, transient unilateral weakness or numbness or visual disturbances ('flashing lights'). Patients will typically want to lie down in a dark room during attacks. Treatment is with simple analgesics and triptans. Prophylaxis is with beta-blockers, amitriptyline, pizotifen and some anticonvulsants.

186. E

Subarachnoid haemorrhage – due to bleeding from intracranial vessels into subarachnoid space. Sudden, severe headache ("my worst headache ever") and they may have been some warning bleeds in the preceding few weeks ('sentinel bleeds'). Meningism (neck stiffness and photophobia) may develop within a few hours and focal neurological symptoms may also develop if the bleed is significant.

187. E

This is from the SCOFF eating disorders questionnaire.

188. C

Obsessive compulsive disorder is a common mental health problem where:

- the obsessive thoughts and/or the compulsive actions should be present on most days for at least two weeks
- there are no passivity symptoms, that is the patient recognises the thoughts and actions as originating from within themselves
- obsessive thoughts and compulsive actions have been unsuccessfully resisted in the past
- the thoughts and actions are unpleasant, if only because of their continual repetition

1–2% of the population have OCD. People at higher risk are those with depression, anxiety, alcohol or substance abuse, eating disorders. Screening questions are:

- Do you wash or clean a lot
- Do you check things a lot
- Do your daily activities take a long time to finish
- Is there any thought that keeps bothering you that you'd like to get rid of but can't?
- Are you concerned about putting things in a special order or are you very upset by mess?
- Do these problems trouble you?

Management is with patient education, CBT and medication. For more information see the NICE quick reference guide at http://www.nice.org.uk/nicemedia/pdf/CG031quickrefguide.pdf

189. D

190. E

191. A

192. F

193. H

Please refer to NICE guidance on management of dyspepsia (2004)

Reference: h ttp://guidance.nice.org.uk/CG17/QuickRefGuide/pdf/English

194. D

195. E

196. A

197. H

198. G

199. C

In swan neck deformity there is hyperextension at the proximal interphalangeal joint (PIP) and flexion at the distal interphalangeal joint (DIP). It occurs in rheumatoid arthritis.

In a boutonniere deformity the PIP is in flexion and the DIP is in hyperextension. It also occurs in rheumatoid arthritis. It results from central slip of the extensor.

200. B

0.5 mg x 20 kg three times a day (tds) = 10 mg tds. These kind of calculations often come up so make sure that you can do them.

Subject Index

Copyright Permission List

Figure 1	Hypertension figure	Permission from NICE
Figure 2	Eczema herpeticum	Differential diagnosis in dermatology
Figure 3	Malignant melanoma	Differential diagnosis in dermatology
Figure 4	L'Abbe plot	Original drawing
Figure 5	Mild acne	Original picture
Figure 6	Management of fibroids	Permission from NICE
Figure 7	Genetic tree	Original drawing
Figure 8	Rhinophyma	Differential diagnosis in dermatology
Figure 9	General practice consultation	Original drawing
Graph 1	Positive skewed distribution	Original drawing
Figure 10	Acne rosacea	Differential diagnosis in dermatology
Figure 11	Sign figure	Original drawing
Table 1	Liver function tests	Original table
Table 2	Full blood count results	Original table
Table 3	Vaginal discharge	Permission from DFSRH
Figure 12	Guttate psoriasis	Differential diagnosis in dermatology
Figure 13	Bell's palsy	Original drawing
Figure 14	SIGN figure	Original drawing
Figure 15	MRI report	Original figure
Figure 16	Meningococcal septicaemia	Differential diagnosis in dermatology
Figure 17	Audit cycle	Original drawing
Figure 18	Horner's syndrome	Lecture notes Ophthalmology
Figure 19	Orbital cellulitis	Lecture notes Ophthalmology
Figure 20	Stages of addiction	Original drawing
Figure 21	Central retinal vein occlusion	Lecture notes ophthalmology
Figure 22	Cholesteatoma	Wikimedia commons
Table 4	Chronic kidney disease	Permission from NICE
Figure 23	Retinal artery occlusion	Lecture notes ophthalmology
Figure 24	LARCs	Permission from NICE
Figure 25	Pyoderma gangrenosum	Differential diagnosis in dermatology
Figure 26	Forest plot	Original drawing
Figure 27	Audiogram	Original drawing
Figure 28	CMV retinitis	Lecture notes ophthalmology

More Titles in the Progressing Your Medical Career Series

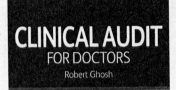

CLINICAL AUDIT
FOR DOCTORS
Robert Ghosh

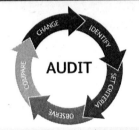

September 2009

160 pages

Paperback

978-1-9068390-1-7

£19.99

develop
medica

Not sure where to start with your clinical audit? Would you like to know how to perform the ideal clinical audit?

It is well recognised that clinical audit is a fundamental tool to maintain high standards of clinical excellence within healthcare. It is therefore important that doctors of all grades of seniority have a clear understanding of what exactly clinical audit is, how to conduct effective clinical audit and how the results contribute to clinical excellence.

'Clinical Audit for Doctors' has been written by doctors for doctors. The target audience ranges widely from medical students to Consultants. It provides step-by-step guidance through the entire clinical audit process, from initial conception to the completion of the clinical audit loop. Through following the clear and concise advice and guidance laid down in this book readers will:

- Learn how involvement in clinical audit can advance your career

- Understand the context clinical audit plays in maintaining clinical excellence as part of clinical governance

- Become clear on how to gain involvement in clinical audit

- Learn how to design, conduct, analyse and present your clinical audit

- Be familiar with the step-by-step instructions on how to design and perform effective clinical audit

This engaging and easy to use book will provide you with the knowledge and skills required to achieve clinical effectiveness through clinical audit.